Improving Health Care Quality: Case Studies with JMP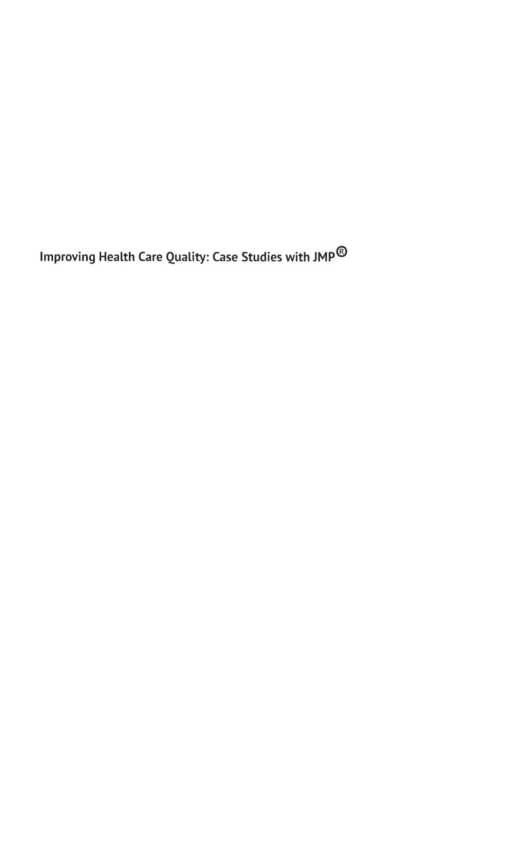

Improving Health Care Quality: Case Studies with JMP®

Mary Ann Shifflet
University of Southern Indiana

Cecilia Martinez
Clarkson University

Jane Oppenlander
Clarkson University

Shirley Shmerling
University of Massachusetts, Amherst

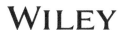

Registered Office
John Wiley & Sons, Inc., 111 River Street, Hoboken, NJ 07030, USA

Editorial Office
111 River Street, Hoboken, NJ 07030, USA

For details of our global editorial offices, customer services, and more information about Wiley products visit us at www.wiley.com.

Wiley also publishes its books in a variety of electronic formats and by print-on-demand. Some content that appears in standard print versions of this book may not be available in other formats.

Library of Congress Cataloging-in-Publication Data

Names: Shifflet, Mary Ann, 1956- author. | Martinez, Cecilia, 1979- author.
 | Oppenlander, Jane, author. | Shmerling, Shirley, 1961- author.
Title: Improving health care quality : case studies with JMP / Mary Ann
 Shifflet, Cecilia Martinez, Jane Oppenlander, Shirley Shmerling.
Description: Hoboken, NJ : Wiley, [2020] | Includes bibliographical
 references and index.
Identifiers: LCCN 2019057873 (print) | LCCN 2019057874 (ebook) | ISBN
 9781119604617 (hardback) | ISBN 9781119604648 (adobe pdf) | ISBN
 9781119604679 (epub)
Subjects: MESH: Quality Improvement | Quality Assurance, Health
 Care–methods | Models, Statistical | Data Analysis | Outcome and
 Process Assessment, Health Care–methods | United States | Case Reports
Classification: LCC RA418 (print) | LCC RA418 (ebook) | NLM W 84.4 AA1 |
 DDC 362.1–dc23
LC record available at https://lccn.loc.gov/2019057873
LC ebook record available at https://lccn.loc.gov/2019057874

Cover Design: Wiley
Cover Image: © Baac3nes/Getty Images

Set in 9.5/12.5pt STIXTwoText by SPi Global, Chennai, India

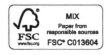

To my husband, Mark, and sons David, Michael and Robert   Mary Ann Shifflet

To my daughter, Anna Victoria   Cecilia Martinez

To my family and my teachers   Jane Oppenlander

To my husband, Dror, and sons Matan and Adi   Shirley Shmerling

Contents

Foreword

If you cannot be one of the authors, being invited to write the Foreword is perhaps the next best thing!

I say this because, when the idea for this project first came about, I had agreed to be one of the co-authors. I was really excited about being a part of it, and to have the opportunity to contribute to the literature of the use of statistical analysis in improving the quality of healthcare delivery. The energy that Mary Ann, Cecilia, Jane, and Shirley each brought to the early discussions about the book was infectious, and I was eager to get started. Unfortunately, due to life circumstances at the time, I had to make the difficult decision to step away. It is so rewarding to see that the book has now come to fruition, and I believe it will become a great addition to the bookshelves of current and future healthcare leaders alike.

With the increasing focus on value, it is now incumbent on all healthcare professionals – not just those in the Quality department – to find ways of improving the quality of the services we and our organizations deliver. Numerous frameworks and programs such as Lean Six Sigma, High Reliability Organization, and the Institute of Medicine's six domains of health care quality (among others) exist to help identify opportunities and implement meaningful change. These evidence-based approaches provide the necessary structure and process for successfully driving quality improvement results throughout a provider organization and help focus the attention of everyone involved toward the critical work required to attain them.

However, while each of these frameworks can be extremely useful as a guide, it is only through the review and analysis of relevant data that the most impactful opportunities for improvement can be appropriately recognized and addressed, and the success of improvement efforts ultimately measured – which is exactly what this book is designed to help you accomplish. Data literacy is now every healthcare leader's responsibility, and this text will help you learn how to apply the concepts, processes, techniques, and tools required for extracting meaningful and actionable information from your data. And do not worry if you have never before studied statistical analysis (or have but are still intimidated by it!), as everything here is presented in a very easy-to-follow, easy-to-understand manner. The use of JMP® software, which itself is quite easy to use, also facilitates the learning process.

I welcome and encourage every reader to use the information in this book to help make the quality of the care your (or your future) organization delivers the absolute best it can be, and I congratulate each of the authors on creating a fantastic resource for all of us in healthcare who strive every day to achieve this important goal. And who knows... maybe I'll get to join in for the Second Edition!

Eric Stephens, MBA, CAP
Chief Analytics Officer
Nashville General Hospital
Nashville, TN
January 11, 2020

Preface

Electronic health records, medical imaging, cell phones/wearable devices, and all-payer claims databases are a few of the technological advances that supply vast amounts of data to the healthcare industry. This data supports the development of new medical devices and pharmaceuticals, enables healthcare systems to contain costs and improve the delivery of services, and informs the medical decision-making of clinicians and patients. The healthcare industry offers a diversity of opportunities for careers in clinical practice, administration, research and analytics. Increasingly, the healthcare workforce must be able to make use of data to tackle a broad range of problems.

As educators, our job is to prepare students with the skills to enter the workforce and be successful contributors in healthcare and other fields. While the four of us have a diversity of experience and backgrounds, we share a desire to teach statistics and quality improvement in a very practical way. Each of us has made use of case studies in our classrooms and found them an effective way for our students to learn practical analytic skills that are easily transferred to the workplace.

As we began to plan what this book would look like we considered several questions. One, what would we find helpful in teaching our students? Two, what would our students find helpful? Three, what would people who are trying to teach themselves about quality improvement find helpful? Those questions led us to the overarching goal of creating practical, real-life case studies for statistics and quality improvement courses that are targeted toward current and future healthcare professionals. These courses can be part of traditional higher education programs with a healthcare focus at either the undergraduate or graduate level or part of continuing education programs for working professionals. Our goal is to offer a set of cases that would provide instruction on most of the statistical tools needed in healthcare quality improvement. A secondary goal was to make the book broad enough to be useful outside the healthcare arena.

We have made a concerted effort to make these cases user friendly for classroom and online instructors, students being assigned cases for learning or assessment, and the self-directed learner seeking to solve practical problems in the workplace. We intentionally created cases of different lengths and levels of difficulty to meet as many needs as possible.

The use of software is now a part of nearly all statistics and quality improvement classes, but integrating technology into a course is always a tricky proposition. In addition to learning the content, there is the added burden for the students to quickly develop facility with a software tool. A frequent debate among statistics educators is the selection of the appropriate software for a particular course with concern about the need to impart software skills that will be applicable in the workplace. Given the number and diversity of available software packages, we are less concerned with specifically which software is used but rather that students at all levels use SOME software to analyze data. The basic concepts associated with any particular software are readily transferred to another. Our software of choice is JMP®. Together, we have many years of experience using JMP in our classrooms, including in online courses. The book is the outgrowth of a project initiated by JMP to fill a need for more healthcare case studies. The focus of the book is on the quality improvement tools and how they are applied to practical problems. While step-by-step JMP navigation is provided, the material will be useful for those preferring other software tools.

The JMP instructions provided refer to JMP version 14; however, most instructions will be appropriate for previous versions. As new versions of JMP are released, there is always excellent backward compatibility. Although the print book is provided in monocolor, the instructions will have color references that refer to items particular to the JMP user interface.

It is our hope that these cases will be engaging for students and instructors and be a valuable resource for the self-directed learner seeking to solve practical problems.

9 March 2020   Jane Oppenlander, Schenectady, NY

Acknowledgments

We would like to thank Mia Stephens of JMP® for bringing a group of strangers together to talk about health care case studies for JMP users. Along with three of the authors, the group included Amy Cohen, Susan Madden, Pat Schaffer, and Eric Stephens. This group brainstormed ideas about how to best meet the needs of health care instructors and professionals who were developing data analysis and JMP skills. The original case structure was the result of these discussions.

A special thanks to Ruth Hummel and Eric Stephens for initial work on the data used in Chapters 3 and 4. Eric also provided invaluable assistance with the data for Chapter 10.

Thanks to Loretta Driskel, Clarkson University, for ideas for graphics.

Thanks to Marilyn Stapleton for her insights into the practice of nursing research along with the nurses of Ellis Medicine for the opportunity to participate in organizational and clinical studies that served as the basis for Chapters 7 and 8.

We would like to give a special thanks to all of our students who helped us improve our teaching over the years, and inspired us to do better every time. We would especially like to thank the students that worked on the ambulatory surgeries and the TJR cases presented here.

We are very appreciative of the two rural hospitals that allowed us to work with them on their process improvement journeys.

A simple thanks is not adequate for our families and friends who supported us during this project. But please know that every word of encouragement or act of kindness helped us to keep going and made our work a pleasure.

Our appreciation for their guidance during this project goes to the editorial staff of Wiley, especially Mindy Okura-Marszycki, Kathleen Santoloci, Blesy Regulas, Linda Christina, and Vishnu Priya. Thanks to everyone who provided feedback at any stage of this project. Your comments and suggestions greatly improved this book.

Acronyms and Synonyms

ASU	Ambulatory Surgical Unit
DMAIC	Define–Measure–Analyze–Improve–Control
DRG	Diagnosis Related Group
EBP	Evidence-Based Practice
ED	Emergency Department
EMS	Emergency Medical Services
ICD	International Classification of Diseases
IRB	Institutional Review Board
MR	Moving Range
OR	Operating Room
PCP	Primary Care Provider
PDCA	Plan–Do–Check–Act
PDSA	Plan–Do–Study–Act
QI	Quality Improvement
SIPOC	Suppliers–Inputs–Process–Output–Customer
SPARCS	Statewide Planning and Research Cooperative System
TJR	Total Joint Replacement
TRIZ	Theory of Inventive Problem Solving
VAS	Visual Analog Scale
VOC	Voice of the consumer
Mean	average
Alternative hypothesis	Research Hypothesis
Significance level	Alpha, Probability of Type I Error
Beta	Probability of Type II Error
Power	1 − Probability of Type II Error

About the Companion Website

This book is accompanied by a companion website:

www.wiley.com/go/shifflet/improvinghealthcarequality1e

Scan this QR code to visit the companion website

The website includes:

Instructor's Site – Figures; Solution manual; Data sets with and without scripts for the Cases and the Exercises

Student's Site – Data sets for the Cases and for the Exercises; Chapter Summaries

1

Introduction

1.1 Key Concepts

Quality improvement (QI) frameworks, Define–Measure–Analyze–Improve–Control (DMAIC), Plan–Do–Check–Act (PDCA), variation, data visualization, statistical tools.

1.2 Quality Improvement in Healthcare

Quality improvement (QI) is an integral component of the healthcare delivery landscape, necessitated by cost escalation and the drive to achieve better individual and population health outcomes. Government and nongovernment organizations at all levels provide resources, strategies, and mandates to achieve global, national, and local health goals. The United States has adopted a national strategy for healthcare quality improvement with three aims: better care, healthy people/healthy communities, and affordable care (Agency for Healthcare Research and Quality 2017). The World Health Organization articulates quality dimensions of effectiveness, efficiency, accessibility, patient-centered, equity, and safety that are applicable to all countries for improving health systems (World Health Organization 2006).

Quality improvement can be defined as the use of a continuous and systematic approach to achieve measurable improvement in healthcare delivery and individual and population health outcomes. Adopting a culture of quality improvement in a healthcare organization can lead to increased efficiency and productivity, better patient and employee satisfaction, the ability to retain and attract high-performing employees, better clinical outcomes, and reduced errors, risks, and costs. Quality improvement should be practiced continuously at all levels and functions of

Improving Health Care Quality: Case Studies with JMP®, First Edition.
Mary Ann Shifflet, Cecilia Martinez, Jane Oppenlander, and Shirley Shmerling.
© 2020 John Wiley & Sons, Inc. Published 2020 by John Wiley & Sons, Inc.
Books Companion site:www.wiley.com/go/shifflet/improvinghealthcarequality1e

an organization. Additional information on quality improvement can be found at the websites of the American Society for Quality and the Institute for Healthcare Improvement.

There are a number of related activities found in healthcare delivery (and beyond) that differ from quality improvement. Quality assurance is a periodic, systematic review of a process to identify and correct errors and ascertain whether standards are being met. Quality improvement and quality assurance both focus on existing systems and processes, with quality improvement programs being driven from within the organization and quality assurance being driven by external organizations (e.g. government and accrediting agencies). Research activity can be found in healthcare organizations, but the emphasis is on attaining knowledge that supports the development of new interventions, products, systems, and processes. Quality improvement, quality assurance, and research share many methodologies and tools; the statistical tools presented in this book focus on quality improvement applications, but can also be used in research and quality assurance.

1.3 Understanding Variability: The Key to QI

Quality improvement can be realized by measurable reductions in cost, errors, or risk, improved health indicators for individuals and populations, and increased patient satisfaction. Healthcare systems and processes are subject to variation due to factors such as the inherent differences in patients, operational practices and procedures, clinician skill and training, and facilities and equipment. Improvements can be made by reducing variation. For example, hospitalized patient satisfaction can be raised and food waste reduced when meals are delivered as scheduled. Achieving improvement requires identifying and understanding the many sources of variation that can affect process performance. For example, timely hospital patient discharge can be affected by variations in staffing levels, pharmacy fulfillment times, demand for beds, etc.

A key step in quality improvement is to create a map or diagram that shows the sequence of the main process steps. Figure 1.1 shows a high-level process map for the preoperative total joint replacement (TJR) process, which will be the subject

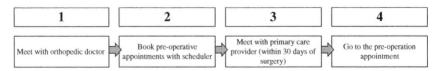

Figure 1.1 Process map for the preoperative total joint replacement.

of three chapters of this book that illustrate the lifecycle of a process improvement initiative.

Such process maps are useful for bounding the scope of the project. Process maps with more detail are good for identifying sources of variability and whether or not these sources of variation are controllable by the organization. Understanding which variability sources are controllable and which are not helps in defining potential improvement actions that an organization can undertake. For example, in Figure 1.1, process step 3 (when the patient meets with the primary care provider), is mostly outside of the control of the hospital, whereas process step 2 (book preoperative appointment) can be changed and is more likely to yield process improvements because patients' preoperative appointment scheduling takes place at the orthopedic clinic.

Sources of variation are also classified as common-cause or special-cause. Common cause variation is inherent in the process and reducing this type of variation, requires a change in the process itself. For example, the variation in the time between process steps 2 (preoperative appointment) and 3 (the preoperative clearance) is between two and four days for knee or hip replacements and seems to be reasonable variation for this part of the process. As such, this would be considered common cause variation. However, the variation in the time between the preoperative appointment and the preoperative clearance can be as high as 40 business days. This unusual variation is attributed to special cause, which arises from unusual circumstances. The variability for the Conformis-brand prosthetic knee replacement process is explained by additional preoperative steps, which not only require extra studies such an magnetic resonance imaging (MRI) but also the fabrication of a prosthetic by a vendor. If there is a problem with the prosthetic, the process takes longer than expected. This special circumstance leads to longer elapsed times than usual, and hence greater process variability that is outside the control of the clinic, adversely affecting the process performance. Identifying variation as either common-cause or special-cause can assist in developing and prioritizing potential improvement actions. In this casebook, we present tools for assessing variability both graphically and numerically. Data visualization and data slicing (or subgrouping) are powerful methods for identifying and quantifying process variation. Additional discussion on variability in the context of quality improvement can be found in Deming (1986) and Hoerl and Snee (2012).

1.4 Quality Improvement Frameworks

Establishing a quality culture requires an ongoing focus on quality throughout an organization, along with a framework and a set of tools for identifying, making, and maintaining improvements. These frameworks serve as a common approach within an organization, enabling project teams to undertake improvement initiatives in a systematic way using a well-defined series of steps. A key component of quality improvement is data collection and analysis to assess process performance. Thus, statistical tools play a key role. Nonstatistical tools, such as brainstorming and process mapping, also have an important role in quality improvement initiatives, particularly in the early stages. There are a number of different frameworks that can be adopted; we will provide a brief overview of two of the most commonly used frameworks.

1.4.1 Define–Measure–Analyze–Improve–Control (DMAIC)

The DMAIC framework is a systematic approach to quality improvement applied in Six Sigma programs. The American Society for Quality (ASQ 2019), defines Six Sigma as "a method that provides organizations tools to improve the capability of their business processes." The DMAIC cycle begins with the Define phase where a team is assembled to develop a project charter that describes the process to be improved and the objectives of the initiative. During this phase, requirements and improvement opportunities are elicited from stakeholders. A clear problem statement is a central part of the project charter. In the Measure phase, a process or value stream map is created to provide stakeholders with a common understanding of how the process operates and serves as the basis for generating improvement ideas. Process performance indicators are also identified, such as delay times and errors. In the Analyze step, the process and associated data are examined to discover potential sources of variation or error. During the Improve phase, process changes that will reduce or eliminate sources of error or variation are developed. Once process changes have demonstrated their effectiveness, they are implemented. Finally, the Control phase puts in place monitoring systems, such as control charts, to ensure that the quality improvements are maintained over time.

The TJR project, parts of which are described in Chapters 12–14, employed the DMAIC framework. Statistical tools including process capability analysis, hypothesis tests, box plots, and dot plots were used in each of the various steps of the process. Insights gained from these tools were critical for the identification of the root cause of the unnecessary process delays. Taken together, in the Improve stage, process root cause countermeasures were brainstormed, solutions designed and evaluated, and pilot testing took place to measure the effectiveness of the solution before its full implementation. In the Control stage, the process elapsed time was monitored in order to maintain the improvements.

1.4.2 Plan–Do–Check–Act (PDCA)

The PDCA framework, synonymous with the Plan–Do–Study–Act framework, is frequently applied to develop and test a quality improvement idea. In the Plan phase, a plan is developed to see if a process change idea will yield a desired improvement. This phase includes developing a problem statement and identifying data to collect to evaluate the change. During the Do phase, the change is implemented as specified in the plan, usually on a small scale. The Check phase evaluates the change using data collected in the Do phase. Finally, in the Act phase, a change that demonstrates significant improvement is deployed as appropriate throughout the organization. If the change does not produce the desired effects, it may be modified and retested or discarded.

As an example, nurses in a hospital wanted to reduce the severity of injuries associated with patient falls. They initiated a PDCA cycle to experiment with fall mats placed next to a patient's bed. They developed a plan to acquire and test the fall mats on a single unit. This change reduced the severity of injuries associated with falls and was adopted on a hospital-wide basis. PDCA initiatives are often conducted sequentially devising, testing, and deploying a series of process changes.

1.4.3 Choosing a Framework

Often, the DMAIC or the PDCA framework is seen as THE framework for quality improvement. While it is good for an organization to have a framework that they typically employ, there should also be a recognition of other frameworks and tools that should be used, depending on the problem to be addressed. The difficulty of process improvement efforts is not the lack of improvement or analysis approaches but matching the right approach to the problem under study. Figure 1.2 provides a matrix for consideration when deciding how to approach a particular type of problem. Typically, process improvement objectives fall into three main categories: (i) reduce process errors, (ii) reduce processing time or waiting times, and (iii) increase utilization of resources. Likewise, there can be three difficulty levels of problems: (i) too easy, problems with known root cause/solutions, (ii) just right, focused problems with nonobvious solutions, and (iii) too difficult, complex, and large problems with unknown root causes most likely coming from different sources. Projects that attempt to solve category three problems are typically known for trying to solve "world hunger." This type of project should be narrow-scoped before attempting any improvement effort. Nevertheless, the improvement methodology should match the problem difficulty level and improvement objective. For example, as shown in Figure 1.2, less difficult projects can be approached with Kaizen. Kaizen is a continuous improvement approach that utilizes short, intensive "events" where dedicated teams work to develop and implement incremental improvements. Lean is the term coined by MIT researchers to describe the way Toyota improved their processes by focusing on value-added activities to identify waste and thus streamline processes (Roos et al. 1991). Thereby, lean works well for projects with less complex problems

	Defect reduction/ Elimination	PDCA Kaizen	DMAIC/Six Sigma	Design for Six Sigma TRIZ-robustness
Type of project	Cycle time reduction	Lean Kaizen	Lean Six Sigma/DMAIC	Lean product development
	Resource consumption minimization	Lean for sustainability Kaizen	Six Sigma/DMAIC for sustainability	Lean Six Sigma for sustainability
		Easy	Non-obvious solution	Systemic
			Project difficulty	

Figure 1.2 Framework-type of problem matrix.

and when the primary interest is in minimizing time and reducing wasteful activities. For nonobvious solution projects, more analysis is often required; in particular, Six Sigma/DMAIC is well suited for minimizing errors. Lean Six Sigma lies at the intersection of these two process improvement objectives, and for more complex problems, process methodologies that look into the redesign of products, processes, and sustainability of resources are better suited for systemic problems such as design for Six Sigma (DFSS).

There are other methodologies used when designing new products such as TRIZ, which is a Russian acronym from "Theory of Inventive Problem Solving," which is based on universal principles of creativity and invention for the design of innovative solutions to design problems (Altshuller 1999). Last, the concept of robustness is also used when solving complex design problems where the objective is to reduce variability in the performance of a product by making improvements in the product design. While these latter approaches originated in the manufacturing sector, these can also be applied to healthcare by focusing on the process or products used necessary for providing patient care. These quality improvement approaches, however, are beyond the scope of this casebook.

1.5 Statistical Tools for Quality Improvement

The use of data and measurement is key to the quality improvement philosophy. Therefore, data collection and analysis tools play an important role in improvement initiatives. The process of applying statistical tools to a quality improvement initiative begins with collecting data that will address the question posed. Generating pertinent and reliable data forms the basis for analysis that guides process changes. The application of formal methodologies in study, experiment, and survey design help assure that the data collected meets the needs of a quality initiative.

Once data has been acquired, a variety of data cleaning techniques, such as subsetting, recoding, or formatting may be needed prior to analysis. An important part of data preparation is making sure variable definitions are clearly understood. Data dictionaries accompany many databases and should be consulted for such definitions. Once the data is ready for analysis, the next step is to become familiar with the data through the use of descriptive statistics and visualizations. These initial data summaries are invaluable to help the analyst identify data anomalies, missing data patterns, outliers, time trends, and patterns of variation. They also assist the analyst in identifying additional statistical analyses that may prove useful in better understanding process performance. Figure 1.3 shows the data analysis process in relation to the DMAIC and PDCA frameworks.

In each of these analysis steps, there are a number of statistical and data management tools that can be applied. For example, hypothesis testing may be needed to ascertain if there are significant differences between average wait times of two different urgent care facilities within the same healthcare network. Data visualization is an integral part of the statistical analysis process. The statistical tools presented in this casebook are those most commonly applied in quality improvement. Additional detail on these tools and other statistical analysis techniques can be found in Babbie (2015), Hoerl and Snee (2012), Polit (2010), and Rosner (2015).

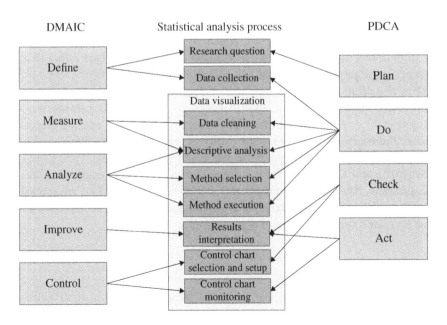

Figure 1.3 Statistical analysis process in QI framework.

1.5.1 Data Visualization

Data visualization plays an important role in quality improvement, as can be seen in Figure 1.3. Once data has been collected, visualizations are useful in the data cleaning process, for assessing variation, in understanding relationships between variables, and for monitoring key process indicators.

Univariate graphs such as histograms and box plots aid in identifying data anomalies, such as transcription errors or misspellings in character fields. These graphs also familiarize the analyst with the distribution of the observations. Outliers are easily seen in histograms and box plots. Outliers may be legitimate, but unusual values of a process or they may be errors that require either correction or removal from the data set. Careful study of outliers may lead to insights that benefit the quality initiative. A control chart, which will be described in more detail later, is another type of univariate graph used to monitor process performance over time.

Bivariate plots, such as scatterplots and run charts allow analysts to detect patterns of variation and time trends. They are also helpful to the analyst in choosing an appropriate form for a statistical model to quantify the relationship between two variables. Multivariate graphs such as bubble plots and scatterplot matrices are effective for displaying three or more variables. Maps are another valuable way to visualize geographic data. JMP®'s Graph Builder offers many options for creating multivariate graphs and implements the data visualization technique of "small multiples" (Tufte 2001). This method displays multiple variables using similar graphs with the same axis scales sequenced over one or two other variables. Small multiples allow the observer to focus on changes in the data rather than changes in the graphical elements.

Data visualizations are easily understood by participants in quality improvement projects and facilitate evaluation of process performance. They are also powerful tools for communicating with management, stakeholders, and the general public. There are a number of principles and best practices to create effective visualizations. The reader is referred to the works of Cleveland (1994), Tufte (2001), Few (2012), and Knaflic (2015) for more guidance on creating compelling data visualizations. The cases presented here illustrate how visualizations are applied in various phases of the DMAIC process and provide step-by-step instructions for how to create a variety of different types of graphs.

1.5.2 Subgrouping Data

Examining data in subgroups, also known as "slicing" the data, or stratification can help project teams discover opportunities for process change. For example, analyzing the time required for nurses to respond to a patient call by shift may identify needed changes to staffing levels to improve patient satisfaction. JMP provides many features that facilitate data slicing, such as the Data Filter, Graph Builder, and Tabulate. Data subgrouping was crucial in the preoperative TJR process improvement effort. Even though the main steps of the preoperative TJR process are the same regardless of the type of implant, the improvement team discovered that there were some extra steps for a particular kind of knee implant. This stratification led the team to analyze these processes separately. Indeed, this data slicing allowed the improvement team to run comparative studies that facilitated the identification of the root cause of the problem as discussed in Chapters 13 and 14.

1.5.3 Control Charts

In practice, process changes are most effective right after they are implemented when awareness is high, but over time, these changes may not be sustained. Control charts are a key tool for monitoring quality improvements to be sure that the desired effect is maintained over time. They track key process variables and alert the user when something has changed in the process performance.

An important feature of control charts is that they display the region corresponding to the expected variability (common cause variation) of a process indicator when it is operating normally (i.e. in control). Observations lying outside of this region alert the user that the process has changed and action should be taken to understand what has changed and deploy any needed corrective actions. There are different types of control charts that depend on the measurement level of the process variable. "Variables" charts are for those variables measured on a continuous scale. "Attribute" charts apply to count measurements, such as number of errors per insurance claim. Figure 1.4 shows some of the commonly applied attribute and variables charts.

Attributes are counts, classified as either defectives or defects. A defective is an item that does not meet the requirements, while defects are the number of non-conformances per item. For example, consider the process of hospital bills being audited periodically. If a bill contains an error, it would be considered defective, and the count of all defective bills during the audit period would be appropriately monitored by P- or NP-charts, depending on whether the number of bills audited in each period is variable or fixed, respectively. In contrast, if the auditors count the number of errors on each bill, then U- and C-charts are applicable, again depending on whether the number of bills audited in each period is variable or fixed, respectively.

A process variable that is continuous is typically monitored using two charts, one to track the process average and one to track the variation. The I–MR chart combination (in JMP referred to as IR) allows a process to be monitored when there

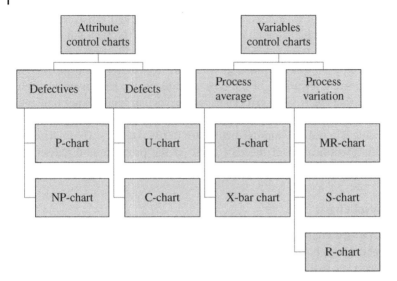

Figure 1.4 Types of control charts.

is only one observation per unit time. For example, an emergency department monitoring the number of hours they are not accepting incoming ambulances (ambulance diversion) would employ I- and MR-charts. X-bar and either an S- or R-chart are applicable when monitoring a process where there are multiple observations per time period, such as the waiting time until a patient completes the intake process in an emergency department. The case "Monitoring Ambulance Diversion Hours" explains the construction and use of I- and MR-control charts. Chapter 11 illustrates several types of control charts. Additional information on control charts can be found in Montgomery (2012).

1.5.4 The Importance of Assumptions

Many of the traditional statistical methods, such as hypothesis testing, have assumptions that must be satisfied for the conclusions to be valid. For example, the assumptions underlying the one sample t-test are that the data are continuous and follow a Normal distribution and were obtained as a simple random sample. Always check the assumptions underlying a statistical method to avoid drawing an erroneous conclusion. For example, constructing a Normal probability plot or performing a Shapiro–Wilks test verifies normality. The degree to which each method is robust to deviations from the assumptions varies. When assumptions are violated, there are often other methods that can be applied. In the case where the normality assumption does not hold in a one sample t-test, the Wilcoxon signed rank test is an alternative. Additional information on dealing with violations of assumptions can be found in Rosner (2015).

1.6   Using this Casebook

This casebook focuses on the use of statistical tools as implemented in JMP for healthcare quality improvement. The cases take a holistic approach to data analysis beginning with background and a specification of the task to be undertaken. The available data is presented and the processing needed to prepare the data for analysis is illustrated. Every analysis begins with descriptive analysis and may be followed by the application of statistical methods, the results of which are interpreted in the case context. Insight and implications from the analysis are then discussed and next actions are suggested. Each case concludes with a table that summarizes the key concepts of statistical analysis, data management, JMP features, and quality tools illustrated. This table is followed by exercises and discussion questions that may be used to master and extend the material presented in the case.

Figure 1.5 shows the correspondence between the case structure and the DMAIC and PDCA frameworks. The key concepts are presented at the beginning of each case and associated with the relevant DMAIC and PDCA steps.

The 13 cases presented in this book cover the most commonly applied statistical tools in quality improvement and show the step-by-step instructions to execute the methods in JMP. The three cases on TJR comprise a complete quality improvement project. Pairs of cases related to a single topic or data set show the application of a sequence of methods, as in the diabetes patient hospitalization

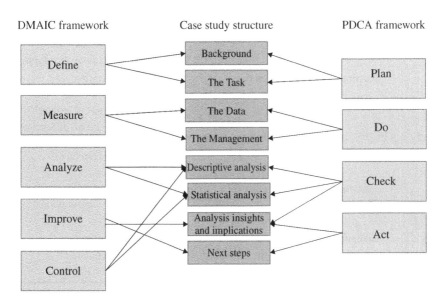

Figure 1.5   Case structure and DMAIC and PDCA frameworks.

data where the first case shows the creation of data visualizations and the second case integrates the data and visualizations in a dashboard (Chapters 3 and 4).

1.7 Summary

Table 1.1 summarizes the statistical tools covered in each of the cases.

Table 1.1 Summary of statistical tools.

Chapter	Title	Statistical tools
2	Improving Patient Satisfaction	Data visualization Descriptive statistics
3	Length of Stay and Readmission for Hospitalized Diabetes Patients	Data visualization Descriptive statistics
4	Identify and Communicate Opportunities for Reducing Hospital Length of Stay Using JMP Dashboards	Data visualization Dashboards
5	Variability in the Cost of Hip Replacement	Data visualization Descriptive statistics Outlier analysis
6	Benchmarking the Cost of Hip Replacement	Descriptive statistics Data visualization Hypothesis test of mean Confidence interval for mean
7	Nursing Survey	Data visualization Descriptive statistics Hypothesis test of proportion Hypothesis test for difference between two proportions Confidence interval for proportion
8	Determining the Sample Size for a Nursing Research Study	Hypothesis testing Sample size determination Power analysis
9	Mapping California Ambulance Diversion	Descriptive statistics Data visualization Geographic mapping

(Continued)

Table 1.1 (Continued)

Chapter	Title	Statistical tools
10	Monitoring Ambulance Diversion Hours	Descriptive statistics Data visualization IR Control charts
11	Ambulatory Surgery Start TImes	IR Control charts X-bar R charts P charts
12	Pre-Op TJR Process Improvement – Part 1	Data visualization Descriptive statistics Time series
13	Pre-Op TJR Process Improvement – Part 2	Data visualization Descriptive statistics Process capability
14	Pre-Op TJR Process Improvement – Part 3	Data visualization Descriptive statistics Hypothesis test on mean difference Confidence interval on mean difference

1.7.1 Exercises

1. Choose a process that occurs daily in your personal or professional life.
   (a) Draw a process map that shows the steps.
   (b) Identify those steps that have controllable or uncontrollable variation.
   (c) For those steps that are within your control, develop actions that could be taken to improve the process.
2. Consider your travel to work or school. Briefly describe your mode of transportation, route, and duration of the trip. Identify the causes of variability in the time to complete your trip and classify them as either common- or special-cause variation. What actions could you take to reduce your travel time variability?
3. Each US state's health department issues a weekly report during influenza season. Choose a state and select one of the weekly reports during the height of flu season. Evaluate the data visualizations presented in the report. Write a paragraph critiquing the visualizations, commenting on those graphs that were effective and those that were not.
4. Draw a high-level process map for the steps involved in having a routine blood draw done as part of an annual physical exam. Identify the steps that add value

from the patient's perspective and the steps that do not, and the steps that are necessary from the clinical point of view. Identify where in the process interruptions or delays are encountered. Are the causes of delays obvious? Are the bottlenecks that prevent the tasks from flowing continuously easy to identify and eliminate? Use Figure 1.2 to identify the process improvement framework that would be appropriate for this case. Justify your answer and identify what kind of data would also be appropriate to collect to narrow scope the project.

1.7.2 Discussion Questions

1. Search the Internet and find a report or journal article that describes a healthcare quality improvement project. Prepare a brief summary of the project and include the following:
   (a) Describe the process to be improved and the associated problem(s).
   (b) What quality improvement framework was used?
   (c) What variables were used to measure the key aspects of the process?
   (d) What changes were made to the process and who developed these changes?
   (e) Specifically, how much improvement was realized (e.g. cost savings, amount of risk reduction) and what monitoring was done to assure that the improvement was sustained?
2. Research nonstatistical tools that are commonly applied in quality improvement initiatives. Give a brief description of each of these tools and identify the steps in the DMAIC and PDCA frameworks in which they are most applicable.
3. Research and share principles of effective data visualization. Identify visualization techniques that should be avoided.
4. Explore the literature to find other quality improvement frameworks. Discuss how they compare to DMAIC and PDCA.

References

Agency for Healthcare Research and Quality (2017). About the National Quality Strategy. https://www.ahrq.gov/workingforquality/about/index.html (accessed 19 August 2019).

Altshuller, G. (1999). *The Innovation Algorithm - TRIZ, Systematic Innovation and Technical Creativity*, 1e. Technical Innovation Center.

ASQ (2019). Building dashboards to access and share updated reports. https://asq.org/quality-resources/six-sigma (accessed 19 August 2019).

Babbie, E. (2015). *The Practice of Social Research*, 14e. Cengage Learning.

Cleveland, W.S. (1994). *The Elements of Graphing Data*, 2e. Hobart Press.

Deming, W.E. (1986). *Out of the Crisis*, 2e. MIT Press.

Few, S. (2012). *Show me the Numbers: Designing Tables and Graphs to Enlighten*, 2e. Analytics Press.

Hoerl, R. and Snee, R. (2012). *Statistical Thinking: Improving Business Performance*, 2e. Wiley.

Knaflic, C. (2015). *Storytelling with Data: A Data Visualization Guide for Business Professionals*. Wiley.

Montgomery, D.C. (2012). *Statistical Quality Control*, 7e. Wiley.

Polit, D.F. (2010). *Statistics and Data Analysis for Nursing Research*, 2e. Pearson.

Roos, D., Womack, J.P., and Jones, D.T. (1991). *The Machine That Changed the World: The Story of Lean Production*. Harper Perennial.

Rosner, B. (2015). *Fundamentals of Biostatistics*, 8e. Cengage Learning.

Tufte, E.R. (2001). *The Visual Display of Quantitative Information*, 2e. Graphics Press.

World Health Organization (2006). *Quality of care: a process for making strategic choices in health systems*. https://www.who.int/management/quality/assurance/QualityCare_B.Def.pdf (accessed 28 December 2019).

2
Improving Patient Satisfaction

2.1 Key Concepts

Exploratory Data Analysis, Process Improvement.

2.2 DMAIC

A: The tools illustrated in this case are frequently applied in the Analysis step of the Define–Measure–Analyze–Improve–Control (DMAIC) approach to process improvement.

2.3 PDCA

DC: In this case, you will use tools that apply to the Do and Check steps in the Plan–Do–Check–Act (PDCA) process.

2.4 Background

A regional endocrinology specialty office is experiencing a decrease in the number of patients seen on a weekly basis. The office consists of four doctors, a nurse practitioner, two registered nurses (RNs), four licensed practical nurses (LPNs), and five administrative staff members. Among the clinic staff, there is some concern that the decrease in volume is due to patient dissatisfaction.

Improving Health Care Quality: Case Studies with JMP®, First Edition.
Mary Ann Shifflet, Cecilia Martinez, Jane Oppenlander, and Shirley Shmerling.
© 2020 John Wiley & Sons, Inc. Published 2020 by John Wiley & Sons, Inc.
Books Companion site:www.wiley.com/go/shifflet/improvinghealthcarequality1e

2.5 The Task

A team is assembled from among the staff members to investigate potential causes of decreased patient volume. The team has little experience with quality improvement or with data analysis. Developing some statistical thinking skills will be an important part of solving this problem. Statistical thinking involves viewing data and data analysis in the context of the entire process in order to improve the process or solve problems with the process (Hoerl and Snee, 2012).

2.6 The Data: ComplaintData.xlsx and PatientFeedback.jmp

ComplaintData.xlsx contains information on 262 customer complaints received over a three-month period. This complaint data is captured through the specialty office website. Variables in the data set are defined in Table 2.1.

PatientFeedback.jmp contains summary information from patient surveys administered over a three-month period. The variable definitions are given in Table 2.2.

Table 2.1 Variable definitions for complaint data.

Variable	Definition
Date	Date complaint filed
Complaint Type	Reason for complaint

Table 2.2 Variable definitions for patient feedback data.

Variable	Definition
Week	Week 1, 2, …
Percent Would Recommend	Percentage of patients who would recommend this office
Wait	Percentage of patients indicating wait time was acceptable
Respect	Percentage of patients indicating they were treated with respect
Enough Information	Percentage of patients indicating they received enough information from their medical provider at this visit

2.7 Data Management

The team begins by looking at the patient complaint data. Import the data into JMP® using the Excel Import Wizard, as shown in Figure 2.1. The first 15 rows are displayed in Figure 2.2. The total number of complaints is 262, as can be seen in the Rows box in the lower left section of Figure 2.2.

It is always a good idea to begin any analysis by reviewing the data type for each of the variables in the data set. Since the Complaint Type variable is text data, JMP assigns the Nominal modeling type, denoted by the red histogram icon (gray in print) next to the column name in Figure 2.2. When the data is imported Date is assigned the Continuous modeling type, as denoted by the blue triangle icon. Typically, date should be treated as ordinal data and can be changed by clicking on the blue icon (gray in print) next to the variable name in the columns box. Note that Date is stored in JMP with a date format. To see this, right click on the column head for Date in the data table and select **Column Info**.

You can save this file as a JMP data set using **File** > **Save As** ComplaintData.jmp.

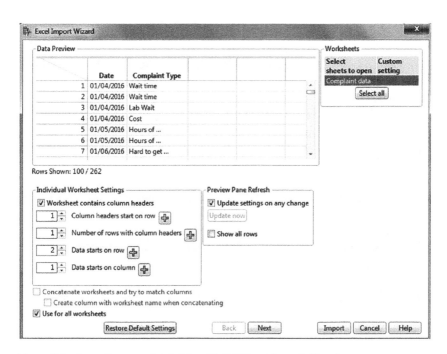

Figure 2.1 Importing complaint data with JMP Excel Import Wizard.
(Navigate to the file; File > Open; Click Import.)

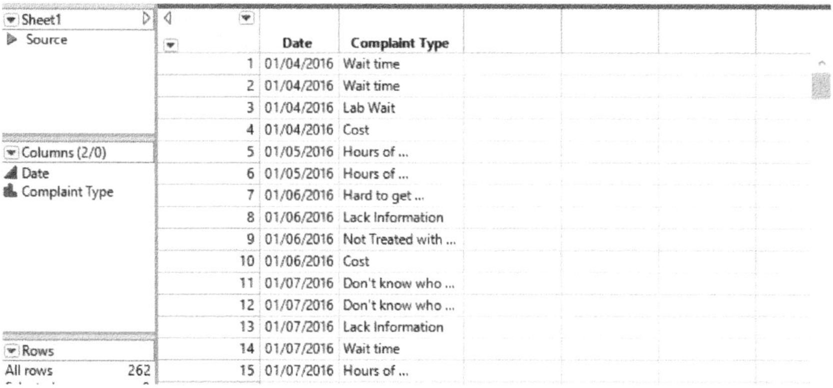

		Date	Complaint Type						
	1	01/04/2016	Wait time						
	2	01/04/2016	Wait time						
	3	01/04/2016	Lab Wait						
	4	01/04/2016	Cost						
	5	01/05/2016	Hours of ...						
	6	01/05/2016	Hours of ...						
	7	01/06/2016	Hard to get ...						
	8	01/06/2016	Lack Information						
	9	01/06/2016	Not Treated with ...						
	10	01/06/2016	Cost						
	11	01/07/2016	Don't know who ...						
	12	01/07/2016	Don't know who ...						
	13	01/07/2016	Lack Information						
	14	01/07/2016	Wait time						
	15	01/07/2016	Hours of ...						

Sheet1
Source
Columns (2/0)
Date
Complaint Type
Rows
All rows 262

Figure 2.2 The complaint data in JMP.

2.8 Analysis

2.8.1 Complaint Data

Since the office has not been in the habit of routinely looking at this data, the group is surprised by the volume of complaints over the last quarter. A Pareto chart (Figure 2.3) is used to summarize the data. A Pareto chart is a special case of a bar chart, where the events are displayed in descending order of frequency of occurrence. So the most frequently occurring event is displayed on the far left and the least frequently occurring event is displayed on the far right of the bar chart. This chart helps the team to prioritize the problems by the most frequently occurring complaint.

You see that there were 262 complaints in the last quarter, and that the top three issues, accounting for 63% of the complaints are Wait Time, Not Treated with Respect, and Lack of Information.

Rather than speculate on causes of negative feedback, the team decides to listen to the "voice of the customer" using a short survey. "Voice of the customer," or VOC, is a term used in quality improvement to refer to the process of obtaining feedback on customer likes, dislikes, and concerns.

Over a three-month period, patients seen in the office are given a short survey as they finish their appointments. The patients are asked the following questions:

- Was the wait time to be seen today acceptable?
- Were you treated with respect by the medical provider and office staff?
- Did you receive enough information from the medical provider?
- Would you recommend this clinic to others?

Distributions

Complaint Type

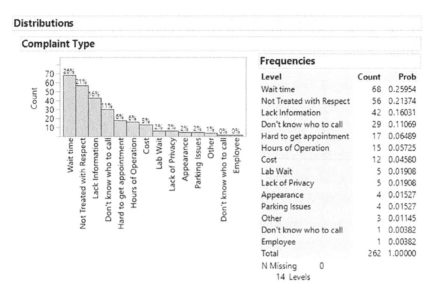

Frequencies

Level	Count	Prob
Wait time	68	0.25954
Not Treated with Respect	56	0.21374
Lack Information	42	0.16031
Don't know who to call	29	0.11069
Hard to get appointment	17	0.06489
Hours of Operation	15	0.05725
Cost	12	0.04580
Lab Wait	5	0.01908
Lack of Privacy	5	0.01908
Appearance	4	0.01527
Parking Issues	4	0.01527
Other	3	0.01145
Don't know who to call	1	0.00382
Employee	1	0.00382
Total	262	1.00000

N Missing   0
14 Levels

Figure 2.3 Pareto chart of complaint data.
(Analyze > Distribution; Select Complaint Type as Y, Click OK; Select Stack under the top red triangle; From the red triangle next to Complaint Type select: Histogram Options > Count Axis and Show Percents; Display Options > Axes on Left and Order By > Count Descending.)

Survey participants used a 7-point Likert scale to indicate their level of agreement with the statement. In the scale used, 1 indicates total disagreement and 7 indicates total agreement. So lower ratings indicate less satisfaction and higher ratings mean the patient is more satisfied.

The team decides to focus on the percentage of satisfied patients. They decide that patients responding with a 6 or a 7 on the Likert scale will be classified as satisfied, while patients responding with at 1–5 will be classified as not satisfied. At the end of the three-month period, for each question, the percentage of satisfied patients is calculated for each week.

2.8.2 Patient Satisfaction Data

The primary measure the team will use to assess patient satisfaction is Percent Would Recommend. The team starts by producing summary statistics for the variable Percent Would Recommend as seen in Figure 2.4.

The mean (average) and the median (middle-most value) are measures of central tendency. It is clear that overall patient satisfaction is much lower than the team expected, with roughly 58% of patients on average reporting that they would recommend the office to others.

	Percent Would Recommend
Mean	57.8
Std Dev	8.9
Median	56.0
Interquartile Range	16.0
Min	42.0
Max	71.0

Figure 2.4 Summary statistics – Percent Would Recommend.
(Analyze > Tabulate; Drag Percent Would Recommend to Drop Zone for Columns; Drag Summary Statistics to Drop Zone for Rows; Click on Change Format box in lower left corner to change decimal format; Choose Use the Same Decimal Format; Choose Fixed Dec, enter 1 under Number of Decimals; Click OK; Click Done to close control panel.)

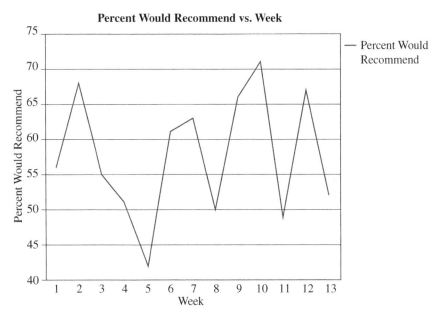

Figure 2.5 Run chart – Percent Would Recommend.
(Graph > Graph Builder; Drag Percent Would Recommend to the Y zone; Drag Week to the X zone; Select the Line icon at the top of the Graph; Right click the y-axis; choose Axis Settings from menu; check box for Major Grid Lines; Click OK to accept axis settings; Click Done to close the Graph Builder control panel.)

The standard deviation (std dev) and the interquartile range (the range of the middle 50% of the values) are measures of spread or variability in patient satisfaction from week to week. The minimum (min) and maximum (max) value, which provide another indication of variability, show that the weekly percentage of satisfied patients ranges from 42% to 71%.

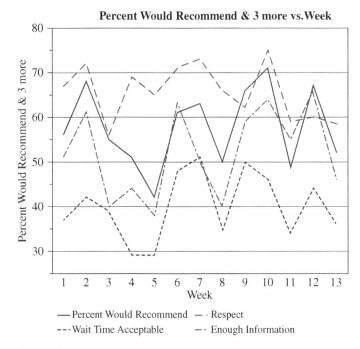

Figure 2.6   Run chart – all four measures.
(From Graph Builder report produced in Figure 2.5, reopen Control Panel by selecting Show Control Panel from red triangle; One at a time, drag each response to the drop zone just inside the *y*-axis; Right click on each response name; select Line Style; click on style choice; Click Done.)

Run charts (Figure 2.5) provide a graphical indication of the central tendency and variability over time. They also allow time-dependent patterns, such as the decrease in Week 5, to be easily detected. (We will revisit whether there are patterns over time in the exercises at the end of this chapter.)

Run charts for the other three measures, along with Percent Would Recommend are given in Figure 2.6. For ease of comparison, the four measures are plotted on the same graph. The values for these variables tend to move together, with the exception of Respect. For example, as Percent Would Recommend goes up Enough Information generally goes up, and as Percent Would Recommend goes down Enough Information generally goes down.

Histograms show the shape, center, and spread of distributions. Histograms for the four responses, generated from the **Distribution** platform, are shown in Figure 2.7. The low values for Percent Would Recommend are shaded, indicating that those rows are selected in the data table. Since the histograms are dynamically linked, the values for the selected rows are highlighted in the other histograms

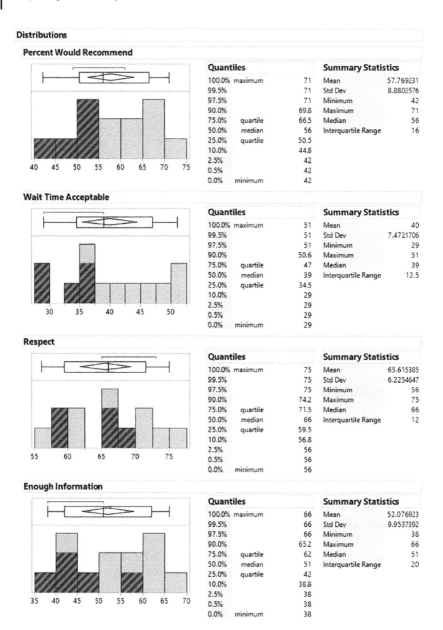

Distributions

Percent Would Recommend

Quantiles			Summary Statistics	
100.0%	maximum	71	Mean	57.769231
99.5%		71	Std Dev	8.8802576
97.5%		71	Minimum	42
90.0%		69.8	Maximum	71
75.0%	quartile	66.5	Median	56
50.0%	median	56	Interquartile Range	16
25.0%	quartile	50.5		
10.0%		44.8		
2.5%		42		
0.5%		42		
0.0%	minimum	42		

Wait Time Acceptable

Quantiles			Summary Statistics	
100.0%	maximum	51	Mean	40
99.5%		51	Std Dev	7.4721706
97.5%		51	Minimum	29
90.0%		50.6	Maximum	51
75.0%	quartile	47	Median	39
50.0%	median	39	Interquartile Range	12.5
25.0%	quartile	34.5		
10.0%		29		
2.5%		29		
0.5%		29		
0.0%	minimum	29		

Respect

Quantiles			Summary Statistics	
100.0%	maximum	75	Mean	65.615385
99.5%		75	Std Dev	6.2254647
97.5%		75	Minimum	56
90.0%		74.2	Maximum	75
75.0%	quartile	71.5	Median	66
50.0%	median	66	Interquartile Range	12
25.0%	quartile	59.5		
10.0%		56.8		
2.5%		56		
0.5%		56		
0.0%	minimum	56		

Enough Information

Quantiles			Summary Statistics	
100.0%	maximum	66	Mean	52.076923
99.5%		66	Std Dev	9.9537392
97.5%		66	Minimum	38
90.0%		65.2	Maximum	66
75.0%	quartile	62	Median	51
50.0%	median	51	Interquartile Range	20
25.0%	quartile	42		
10.0%		38.8		
2.5%		38		
0.5%		38		
0.0%	minimum	38		

Figure 2.7 Distributions with dynamic linking.
(Analyze > Distribution; Drag all four variables to Y, Columns; click OK; Select Stack from red triangle next to Distributions; Hold shift key and click on each of the lowest bars for Percent Would Recommend.)

	Percent Would Recommend	Wait Time Acceptable	Respect	Enough Information
Mean	57.8	40.0	65.6	52.1
Std Dev	8.9	7.5	0.2	10.0
Median	56.0	39.0	66.0	51.0
Interquartile Range	16.0	12.5	12.0	20.0
Min	42.0	20.0	56.0	38.0
Max	71.0	51.0	75.0	66.0

Figure 2.8   Summary statistics – all four measures.
(From Tabulate report produced in Figure 2.4, select Show Control Panel from red triangle; Drag each variable, one at a time, to the Drop Zone for Columns area next to Percent Would Recommend; Click Done to close control panel again.)

as well. This confirms that low values for Percent Would Recommend generally correspond to low values for the other variables (except Respect).

Along with the histograms, the **Distribution** platform provides summary statistics for each of the measures (see Figure 2.7). However, a more effective way to compare the summary statistics for the four variables is to use **Tabulate**, as shown in Figure 2.8.

These measures confirm some of what the team learned from the patient complaint data. A low percentage of patients respond that the wait time is acceptable and that they are given enough information from the provider. These are clearly two important areas that the team must address.

To better understand whether long wait times and not receiving enough information might be related to low recommendations, the team looks at the correlations among the four variables. A table of correlations, along with the corresponding scatterplot matrix is shown in Figure 2.9.

A correlation is a numeric measure of the strength of the linear relationship between two numeric variables. A correlation value close to one indicates a strong positive relationship, a value close to negative one indicates a strong negative relationship, and a value close to zero indicates a weak or no relationship. While not proving causation, a high correlation can, in some cases, be an indicator of a potential cause-and-effect relationship.

The scatterplot matrix (bottom of Figure 2.9) provides a visual representation of the relationships between pairs of variables. The graphs in the first row of the matrix represent the relationships between Percent Would Recommend and each of the other measures. The tighter (narrower) the ellipses, the stronger the correlation.

The high correlations between Acceptable Wait Time and Percent Would Recommend (0.85) and between Enough Information and Percent Would Recommend (0.82) suggest potential to improve Percent Would Recommend by solving these two problems.

Multivariate

Correlations

	Percent Would Recommend	Wait Time Acceptable	Respect	Enough Information
Percent Would Recommend	1.0000	0.8452	0.4128	0.8242
Wait Time Acceptable	0.8452	1.0000	0.3189	0.6779
Respect	0.4128	0.3189	1.0000	0.3058
Enough Information	0.8242	0.6779	0.3058	1.0000

The correlations are estimated by Row-wise method.

Scatterplot Matrix

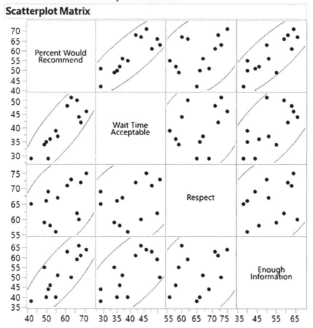

Figure 2.9 Correlations and Scatterplot Matrix.
(Analyze > Multivariate Methods > Multivariate; Select all variables of interest as Y, Columns; Click OK.)

2.9 Summary

2.9.1 Statistical Insights

The process improvement team has used historical data to understand the most frequently occurring complaints to begin to uncover why patient volume has decreased. The most commonly occurring complaints are unacceptable wait times, not being treated with respect, and lack of information from the medical provider.

Based on the complaint data, a survey was conducted with current patients. The survey indicated that low Percent Would Recommend values were associated with low values of both Wait Time and Enough Information. The association could be an indicator of cause and effect.

2.9.2   Implications and Next Steps

Based on the survey data analysis, the team will assemble to brainstorm ways to improve wait time and the information provided to patients by the provider.

Process improvement tools such as cause-and-effect diagrams will be used.

From these efforts, changes will be implemented and the survey data will continue to be used to monitor the process performance to determine if the changes have been effective.

The primary measure of interest is the patient volume which will also be monitored for improvement and sustainability.

2.9.3   Summary of Tools and JMP Features

Statistical methods tools	Data management concepts	JMP platform features	Quality tools
Data visualization	Import Excel spreadsheet	Graph builder	Pareto chart
–Bar chart			
–Run chart			
–Histogram			
Descriptive statistics		Distribution	Voice of customer
–Summary statistics			
–Correlations			
		Tabulate	Statistical thinking
		Multivariate methods	Brainstorming

2.9.4   Exercises

1. Use the PatientFeedback.jmp data to answer the following questions:
   (a) Is the distribution for Percent Would Recommend symmetric?
   (b) Based on the shape of the distribution for Percent Would Recommend, which measure of centrality, mean, or median, is the most representative? Explain why.

(c) For the run chart in Figure 2.5 (Percent Would Recommend), the default y-axis setting is roughly 40–70%. Why might it make more sense to change the axis to 0–100%?

(d) Recreate the run chart shown in Figure 2.6. Identify the weeks in which Percent Would Recommend was particularly high or low. Are the other variables also high or low? Does this tell you anything about cause and effect?

2. Use the ComplaintData.jmp file to reproduce the Pareto Chart given in Figure 2.3 using the Quality and Process platform instead of the Distribution Platform (Analyze > Quality and Process > Pareto Plot). What are the top five patient complaints? What percentage of all complaints do the top five account for?

3. Open the Fitness.jmp data set in the JMP Sample Data directory (Help > Sample Data Library). Answer the following questions:

(a) Create a scatterplot matrix, and find the correlations among the continuous variables following the directions in the case.

(b) Which pair of variables has the strongest positive correlation (and what is the value)?

(c) Which pair of variables has the strongest negative correlation (and what is the value)?

(d) What does the negative correlation indicate?

4. The data set ComplaintDataEx.jmp contains data collected for a three-month period after steps were taken to address the top two complaints.

(a) Create a Pareto Plot for Complaint Type. Was there improvement in Wait Time? Are there other key issues that need to be addressed?

(b) Create a new formula column for day of the week. Create both a graph and a tabular summary of complaints by day of the week. Describe what you learn. Are there more complaints on some days than others? Do complaint types occur more frequently on some days than on others? How could these issues be addressed?

(c) Create a new formula column for week. Create a run chart for complaints by week. Describe what you observe.

(d) Explore the data using other tools available in JMP. Can we learn anything else from these data?

2.9.5 Discussion Questions

1. The file ComplaintData.jmp contains complaint type and the date of the complaint. This information was downloaded from the specialty office website.

(a) Discuss the quality of this information for understanding customer complaints.

(b) What additional information would be useful?

(c) What information should be captured by the complaint data collection system?

2. The data in the file PatientFeedback.jmp contains summarized satisfaction results based on customer surveys.
   (a) Discuss how these data were collected and summarized.
   (b) From a data collection perspective what would you do differently (if anything)?
   (c) What would you recommend for collecting patient satisfaction information going forward?
3. Discuss the difference between correlation and causation. Specifically, why does correlation not imply causation? Provide at least one example where there is a strong correlation but clearly no evidence of causation.
4. How is causation established? Discuss what actions might be taken to establish causation.
5. In this case, the team has identified some potential causes for poor patient satisfaction ratings. What are potential next steps to address these issues?
6. After changes are implemented to address the issues, how will you verify that the changes made have improved patient satisfaction and patient volume? How will you verify that these issues do not return (i.e. that patients continue to be satisfied and that the number of patients seen does not drop over time)?

Reference

Hoerl, R. and Snee, R. (2012). *Statistical Thinking: Improving Business Performance*, 2e. Wiley.

3

Length of Stay and Readmission for Hospitalized Diabetes Patients

3.1   Key Concepts

Data exploration, data visualization.

3.2   DMAIC

MAI: In this case, you will use tools that apply to the Measure, Analyze, and Improve steps in the Define–Measure–Analyze–Improve–Control (DMAIC) approach to process improvement.

3.3   PDCA

PD: In this case, you will use tools that apply to the Plan and Do steps of the Plan–Do–Check–Act (PDCA) approach.

3.4   Background

Two of the key measures for hospitals in improving efficiency are the average length of stay and the readmission rate. For patients and families, these may seem like measures that are only aimed at cutting costs. However, reducing length of stay can be an important quality measure as well. Reducing the length of the hospital stay reduces the opportunities for adverse events, such as falls and infections, which is especially important for diabetes patients. Hospital readmission rates are indicators not only of quality of care during hospitalization but also an indicator of quality of follow-up care.

Improving Health Care Quality: Case Studies with JMP®, First Edition.
Mary Ann Shifflet, Cecilia Martinez, Jane Oppenlander, and Shirley Shmerling.
© 2020 John Wiley & Sons, Inc. Published 2020 by John Wiley & Sons, Inc.
Books Companion site:www.wiley.com/go/shifflet/improvinghealthcarequality1e

This case uses data obtained from the UC Irvine Machine Learning Repository and basic data visualization tools to identify trends in length of hospital stay and readmission, potential causes of longer stays, and potentially relevant indicators of reduced length of stay and readmissions.

3.5 The Task

You will be using data visualization tools to explore both length of stay and hospital readmission for diabetes patients.

3.6 The Data: HospitalReadmission.jmp

The variables of interest are defined in Table 3.1.

3.7 Data Management

No data management is required for the analysis shown in this case.

Table 3.1 Variable definitions.

Variable	Definition
Year	Year of encounter
Race	African-American, Asian, Caucasian, Hispanic, other
Gender	Female, Male
Age	Age group
time in hospital	Number of days
Readmitted	<30 days, >30 days, not readmitted
Readmit indicator	Yes, No
Diag-Code 1	Primary diagnosis code

3.8 Analysis

One of the first steps in the DMAIC approach to process improvement is to Measure the process. In this case, one of the ways to begin to measure the process is to view the data over time. In doing so, you can answer basic questions such as

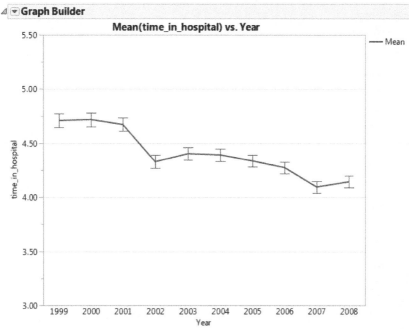

Each error bar is constructed using a 95% confidence interval of the mean.

Figure 3.1 Run chart of time in hospital.
(Click on Graph > Graph Builder; Drag Year to *x*-axis; drag Year to *y*-axis; click on line icon at the top to connect the points; Hover over *y*-axis until hand tool appears; click on axis settings; Select 3.0 as minimum and 5.5 as the maximum with 0.5 increment; choose major grid lines in the upper right box; Select Confidence Interval from drop down Error Bars menu.)

"how is the process currently performing?," and "is the process improving or getting worse?." Figure 3.1 shows the average time in hospital over the 10-year period covered in the data, with 95% confidence intervals on the mean included.

Notice that the average time in hospital decreases a little more than half a day over the 10-year time period. From the hospital point of view, this could be seen as a modest improvement. The confidence intervals take into account the variability in time in hospital as well as the average on a yearly basis. Quantifying the variability is an important aspect of any process improvement project.

In addition to observing the data over time, basic summary distributions give a snapshot of both measures. Figures 3.2 and 3.3 provide distributions for the key measures, time in hospital, and readmitted. Figure 3.2 shows an average time in hospital of 4.4 days, standard deviation of about 3 days, and the histogram illustrates that the majority of patients had a stay of less than 5 days. Over half the

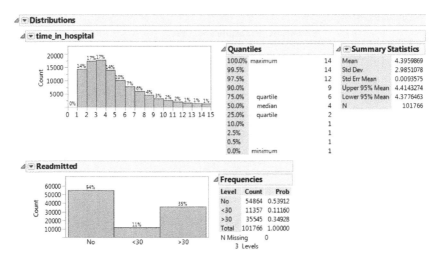

Figure 3.2 Distributions of time in hospital and readmitted.
(Click on Analyze and select Distribution; Drag time in hospital and readmitted to the y box; click OK; Click red triangle next to Distributions and select Stack; For each variable click on red triangle next to variable name and select Histogram options; Choose both Count axis and Show Percents; Under Display options for both variables select Axes on Left; For time in hospital change *x*-axis settings to minimum = 0, maximum = 15, increment = 1 and minor ticks = 0.)

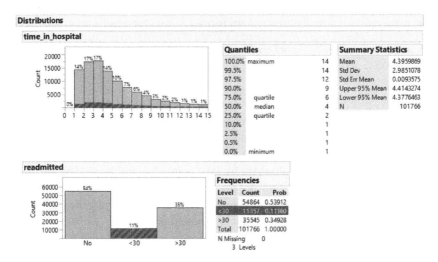

Figure 3.3 Distributions of time in hospital and readmitted with readmit <30 days highlighted.
(Click on <30 bar to view dynamic linking.)

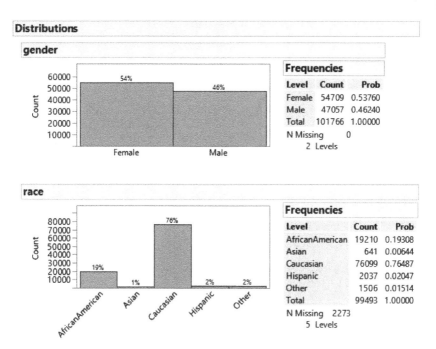

Figure 3.4 Bar charts for gender and race.
(Follow same steps as in Figure 3.2.)

patients were not readmitted to the hospital, and only 11% were readmitted within a month of discharge. Figure 3.3 takes advantage of the dynamic linking of JMP® by highlighting the patients that were admitted within 30 days of discharge. Notice in the time in hospital histogram that the pattern is the same for those patients readmitted soon after discharge as for the overall patient group.

One of the first things to consider in any analysis is the subgroups or demographic groupings in the data. For instance, in this example, looking at things like gender and race may be informative, as one of the focal areas in healthcare quality is equality of access and treatment. Figure 3.4 indicates that about 54% of the subjects are female and 46% are male. We see that the vast majority of these patients are Caucasian, about 20% are African American, and less than 5% of the patients are Asian or Hispanic. The small sample sizes for the Asian and Hispanic groups will make it challenging to evaluate the key measures for those subgroups.

In addition to simply looking at the subgroups, a next step would be looking at the time trends for these subgroups, as seen in Figures 3.5 and 3.6. Figure 3.5 indicates that for both Males and Females, the average time in hospital is decreasing,

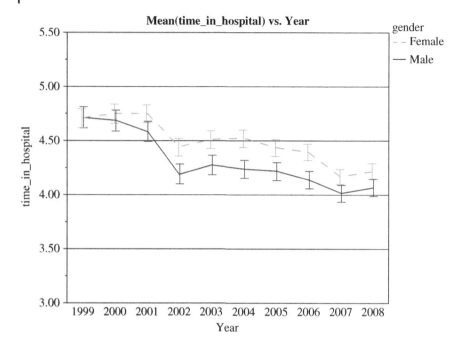

Figure 3.5 Line plot of time in hospital by gender.
(Follow same steps as in Figure 3.1 and drag Gender to Overlay box in upper right corner; Right click on line for Females in legend and change line type.)

but we see that Females have slightly longer average stay than Males – a difference that did not exist at the beginning of the 10-year period. While the difference is not large, it might indicate a place to look for improvement, not only in length of stay but potentially in quality of care as well.

In Figure 3.6, we see some differences between the race categories. Error bars or confidence intervals are not included due to the small sample sizes for some of the subgroups. African Americans tend to have somewhat longer hospital stays on average than other groups. This could be another area to investigate to improve quality of care.

To focus on the two largest Race categories without rerunning analyses, we can take advantage of the JMP dynamic linking by highlighting the two groups in the race histogram. Figure 3.7 illustrates the highlighted bar chart and run chart. We see that the patterns are fairly similar for these two groups, with the

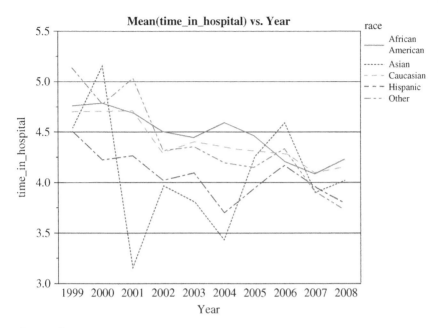

Figure 3.6   Line plot of time in hospital by race.
(Follow same steps as in Figure 3.1 and drag Race to Overlay box in upper right corner;
Change line types by right clicking on lines in legend.)

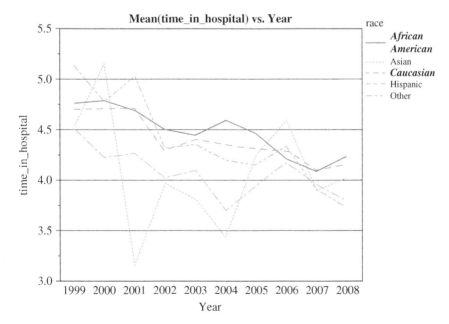

Figure 3.7   Line plot of time in hospital by race with selected categories highlighted.
(From Figure 3.6 hold CTRL key and select African American and Caucasian categories.)

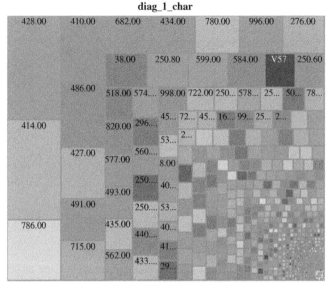
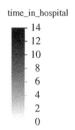

Figure 3.8 Tree map of primary diagnosis and time in hospital.
(Open Graph Builder and drag primary diagnosis code (diag 1 char) to center of graph; Select the treemap icon from the top menu; In the Treemap menu at the left select Squarify as the layout; Right click on the color bar to select color scheme by selecting Gradient; Click on Color Theme to make selection. Theme shown is White to Black Sequential.)

African-American patients typically having only slightly higher average length of stay compared to Caucasian patients.

Another investigation that may be important is to look for groups that typically have a longer stay than others. Using the diagnosis codes and the time in hospital may uncover groups that need some improvement. The codes in this data are International Classification of Diseases (ICD)-9 codes. The ICD coding system is an international system of classifying diseases, procedures, and illnesses. The coding system allows for consistency in recording and thus reasonable comparisons across institutions. A tree map of diagnosis codes with average Time in Hospital color coded is given in Figure 3.8. Use of the squarify option means that the left column and top row are the most frequently seen diagnosis codes. The color indicates the average length of stay, with darker color indicating longer stay. We see the most common primary diagnosis code are 428, 414, and 786, Congestive Heart

Failure, Coronary Atherosclerosis, and Respiratory Abnormality, respectively. The diagnosis with the longest average length of stay is V57, which is a code used for patients receiving rehabilitation services. It is expected that rehabilitation patients will have longer lengths of stay than other patients. Since for insurance purposes, rehabilitation services must be the primary diagnosis, this may not be particularly informative.

3.9 Summary

3.9.1 Statistical Insights

At the beginning of a quality improvement initiative, visualizing the available data familiarizes the analyst with the historical performance of the process and can reveal opportunities for process improvement. Observations made from this analysis:

- On average, women have longer length of stays than men.
- African Americans tend to have higher mean lengths of stay than Caucasians. These two groups comprise 96% of this patient population.
- Short readmission times do not appear to be associated with hospital length of stay.
- Congestive heart failure, coronary atherosclerosis, and respiratory abnormality are the most common primary diagnoses for this patient population.
- The longest average length of stay was experienced by patients receiving rehabilitative services.

3.9.2 Implications and Next Steps

Visualizing data is an easy way to discover patterns and trends in the length of stay and readmission among hospitalized diabetes patients. However, significant differences cannot be established from visualization alone. Methods such as hypothesis testing or statistical modeling are required to establish significance. The graphs presented in this case are static and may not meet the needs of particular inquiries. Creating dashboards allows users to interact with the data and create and share visualizations that address a wide variety of problems. Dashboards are valuable for ongoing performance monitoring, assessing effectiveness of quality initiatives, and searching for possible additional process changes.

3.9.3 Summary of Tools and JMP Features

Statistical methods tools	Data management concepts	JMP platform features	Quality tools
Data visualization		Graph builder	Process variation
–Histogram			
–Bar chart			
–Line plot			
–Tree map			
Descriptive statistics	Value reordering	Distribution	Sources of variation
–Mean			
–Standard Deviation			
		Column properties	Statistical thinking
		–Modeling type	
		–Value ordering	

3.9.4 Exercises

1. The use of "small multiples" is a data visualization technique that allows multi-variate data to be displayed by a series of similar graphs sequenced by categories of another variable. The method was popularized by Edward Tufte. Research small multiples and use Graph Builder to create a visualization of the line graph in Figure 3.7 using small multiples. Discuss the advantages and disadvantages of these two presentations.

2. Recreate the graphs of Figure 3.3 for patients who were not readmitted and for patients that were readmitted >30 days. Prepare the graphs so that they are suitable to include in a report or presentation (for example, use y-axis scales, counts/percentages).

3. Create a visualization that compares the distributions of length of stay by gender.

4. How do the patterns of hospital length of stay and readmission differ by age group? Create visualizations similar to those presented in this case and prepare two to three presentation slides that summarize your findings.

3.9.5 Discussion Questions

1. What other factors, not available in the data set, might be helpful in finding improvements that would reduce length of hospital stays and readmissions?
2. Search the Internet for articles or studies that report on initiatives to reduce length of stay or readmission for diabetes patients. Summarize your findings and comment on the methods used to achieve improvement.

4

Identify and Communicate Opportunities for Reducing Hospital Length of Stay Using JMP® Dashboards

4.1 Key Concepts

Dashboards, Data Visualization, Effective Communication.

4.2 DMAIC

AC: The tools presented in this case are applicable in the Analyze and Control steps in the Define–Measure–Analyze–Improve–Control (DMAIC) approach to process improvement.

4.3 PDCA

DA: In this case, you will use tools applicable to the Do and Act steps in the Plan–Do–Check–Act (PDCA) approach.

4.4 Background

This case builds on the data visualization case presented in Chapter 3 by creating dashboards that enable investigators to share the visualizations and interact with the data as they search for best practices for treating patients with diabetes while they are hospitalized. Dashboards have become an important part of the business landscape, providing a quick overview of key indicators, such as length of hospital stay and readmission rates. Typically, dashboards are used to share routine analyses with those in the organization who can drive change and improvement.

Improving Health Care Quality: Case Studies with JMP®, First Edition.
Mary Ann Shifflet, Cecilia Martinez, Jane Oppenlander, and Shirley Shmerling.
© 2020 John Wiley & Sons, Inc. Published 2020 by John Wiley & Sons, Inc.
Books Companion site:www.wiley.com/go/shifflet/improvinghealthcarequality1e

Dashboards eliminate the need to conduct analyses every time data is updated. "Process improvement studies are of no value unless the process changes identified by the studies are implemented. This typically requires that the study results be presented to management and others to build support for the proposed changes and obtain the needed resources." (Hoerl and Snee, 2012). For more details on best practices in the use of dashboards see *Performance Dashboards* (Eckerson, 2011).

4.5 The Task

You will be creating JMP dashboards to find and communicate opportunities for reducing time in hospital for diabetes patients. The visualizations created in Chapter 3 will be used to develop the dashboards. Prior to creating the dashboards, you will need to run the analyses discussed in Chapter 3.

4.6 The Data: HospitalReadmission.jmp

The data used in this chapter is the same data used in Chapter 3.

4.7 Data Management

No further data management is needed for this case.

4.8 Analysis

4.8.1 Creating Dashboards with Combine Windows

JMP offers a number of ways to create dashboards. The Dashboard option provides several templates for getting started with a dashboard. However, the easiest way to create a dashboard is to use the Combine Windows feature. This allows users to combine any windows created in JMP. Figure 4.1 is a simple dashboard allowing us to explore whether patients who are released in the shortest amount of time are also the patients readmitted. In other words, are diabetes patients being released from the hospital before they are healthy enough?

Once the windows are combined the result is a fully interactive, editable dashboard. In Figure 4.1, we see that those readmitted in less than 30 days have been highlighted. We see a similar pattern in the distribution of time in hospital for those readmitted quickly compared to the patient group as a whole, indicating little to no association between length of stay and being readmitted quickly.

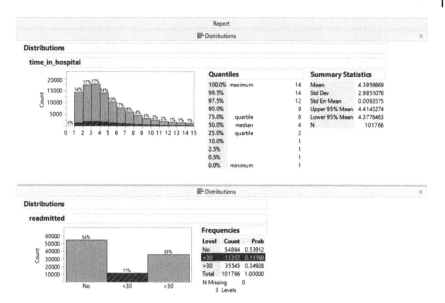

Figure 4.1 Dashboard using combine windows.
(Select Combine Windows from the JMP Window menu; Choose Distribution of time in hospital and Distribution of Readmitted and click OK.)

4.8.2 Creating Dashboards with Dashboard Builder

Prior to launching the dashboard builder, any output that might be used in a dashboard must be created. Follow the instructions from Chapter 3 to create the visual displays necessary to build the dashboards described in this chapter. Once all analyses are run, they are available in the Reports section of the **Dashboard Builder**. The first step in the process of constructing a dashboard is to think about which key measures will be displayed, what analyses will be included, and what format the dashboard will have. The template options in the **Dashboard Builder** are given in Figure 4.2. If the specific panel configuration you are looking for is not available, then select the one closest to your needs. More panels can easily be added to the preset template.

When the dashboard template is selected, available reports are listed in the left column, as seen in Figure 4.3, where the 2×1 Dashboard is selected. Note, the 2×1 template indicates the dashboard will have two panels in one row.

To create the dashboard, drag the appropriate report into the desired panel. To preview the dashboard, click on the red triangle (gray in print) next to Dashboard Builder. Figure 4.4 is the dashboard with time in hospital by year in panel 1 and time in hospital by year for each gender in panel 2.

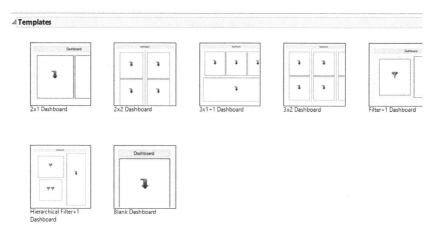

Figure 4.2 Dashboard Builder Templates.
(From the File menu select New > Dashboard.)

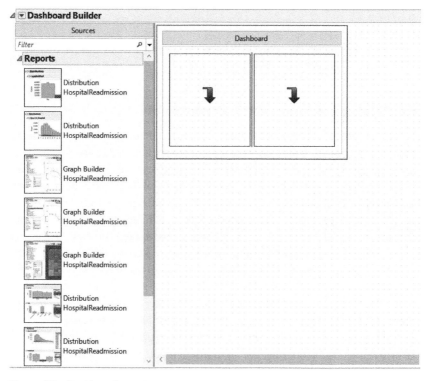

Figure 4.3 Dashboard template.
(Click on the 2 × 1 Template.)

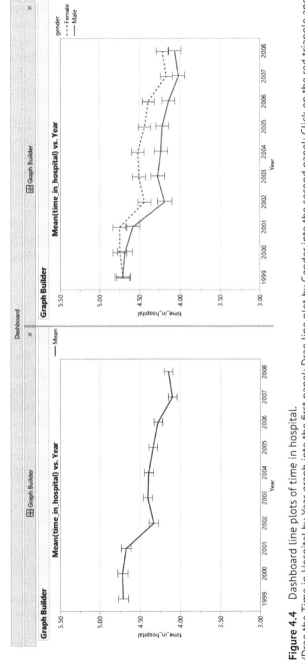

Figure 4.4 Dashboard line plots of time in hospital.
(Drag the Time in Hospital by Year graph into the first panel; Drag line plot by Gender into the second panel; Click on the red triangle and run the dashboard.)

Notice in Figure 4.3 the drag and drop options under Boxes on the left side of the template. A local data filter (for subsetting the data) can be added to the dashboard, a data table can be added, as well as picture files and text boxes. These features will allow for better communication of key information and more interactivity. In addition to adding features to the basic dashboard, additional reports can be inserted, either as additional panels or as tabbed reports within one of the existing panels. Figure 4.5 gives the dashboard with the tabbed report added as well as a logo.

In Figure 4.5, notice that there are two graphs in the second panel. When you preview or run the dashboard, you will be able to switch back and forth between the two reports in the second panel simply by clicking on the tabs at the top of that panel. Both reports are totally interactive, allowing for more detailed investigation of gender and race.

For any dashboard built, there is an option to add a local data filter to provide additional interactivity. Figure 4.6 gives the dashboard from Figure 4.1 filtered by Gender. Figure 4.6a gives the distributions for females, the Figure 4.6b is for males. This allows analysts to investigate differences in time in hospital and readmission rates for males and females.

4.8.3 Saving and Sharing JMP Dashboards

There are several options for saving and sharing dashboards. Save the dashboard file as a jmpappsource if your work is not complete and you would like to come back to that file. Save the dashboard file as a jmpapp file if you would like to share the dashboard with other jmp users in your organization. If the dashboard will have routine use, saving it as an add-in allows for repeated use by individuals when data is updated. Saving as an interactive HTML file or a web report allows for sharing with people who may not have JMP or for embedding the dashboard in a web page. Additional details for saving and sharing dashboards can be found in the webcast in JMP (2019). The instructions for saving and sharing a dashboard are given in Table 4.1.

4.9 Summary

4.9.1 Statistical Insights

The interactivity and filtering capabilities of the dashboard provide a flexible tool that can be used by a variety of personnel to explore and monitor the process.

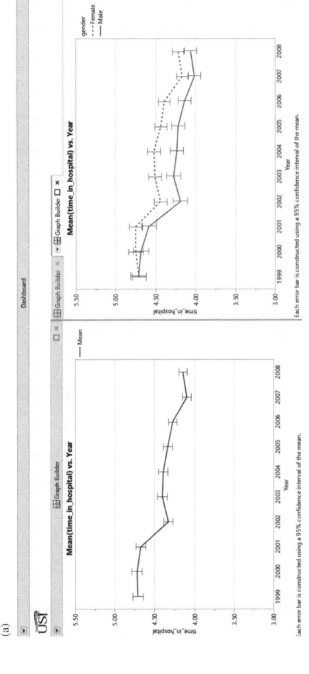

Figure 4.5 2 × 1 dashboard line plots of time in hospital with Tabbed Report, Title, and Logo. Panel (a) gives the run plot for Gender, while Panel (b) gives the run plot for Race. (Drag the Text box to the top of the dashboard and input the title (in this case, the text font was increased in size and bolded); drag the Pict Box to the top of the dashboard and input the picture (in this case a logo); drag the line plot by race into the second panel to create a tabbed panel.)

(b)

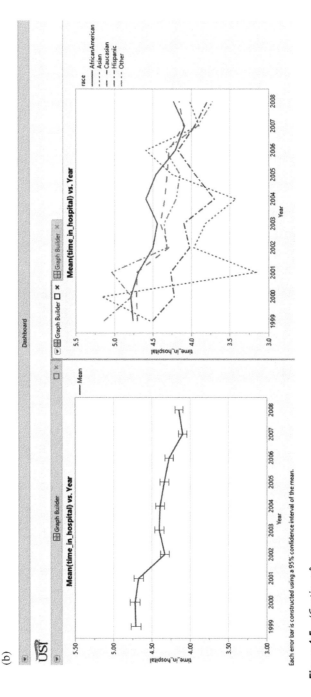

Each error bar is constructed using a 95% confidence interval of the mean.

Figure 4.5 (*Continued*)

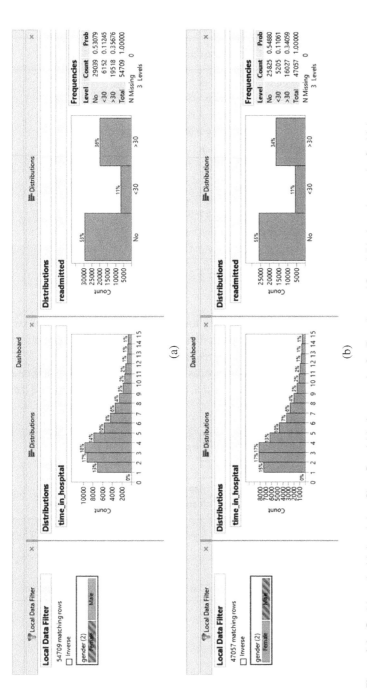

Figure 4.6 Dashboard with local data filter. Panel (a) gives results for Females and Panel (b) gives the results for Males. (Drag the Data Filter box to the left side of the dashboard and run dashboard; In the data filter box, highlight the variable for filtering (in this case Gender) and click Add.)

Table 4.1   Saving and sharing dashboards.

Purpose	File type	Instructions
Working file	jmpappsource	From Dashboard editor: File > Save as > Title
Share	jmpapp	From Dashboard editor: File > Save as > Title.jmpapp
Routine sharing	Add-in	From Dashboard editor: File > Save Script > To Add-in In Add-in menu name the dashboard
Sharing with non-JMP users	Interactive HTML	Run Dashboard File > Save as > HTML
Use in web page	Web report	Run Dashboard File > Publish > Select Appropriate Dashboard

4.9.2   Implications and Next Steps

Creating and deploying dashboards throughout an organization encourages personnel at all organizational levels to use data to evaluate the performance of processes and discover potential process improvements.

The various ways in which JMP dashboards can be saved and shared facilitates wide distribution throughout an organization, thus enhancing the quality and data analysis culture.

4.9.3   Summary of Tools and JMP Features

Statistical methods tools	Data management concepts	JMP platform features	Quality tools
Data visualization		Combine windows	Statistical thinking
–*Histogram*			
–*Line plot*			
		Dashboard builder	Communication

4.9.4 Exercises

1. Recreate the 2 × 1 dashboard developed in this case and then add a report that shows a graph of mean time in hospital by age group.
2. Search the Internet to find an online dashboard.
   (a) Familiarize yourself with the dashboard, its features, and the available data.
   (b) Discuss what insights you gained from using the dashboard.
   (c) Evaluate the usability of the dashboard. What features were particularly useful? What were the limitations of the dashboard?
3. Research best practices in dashboard design and prepare a brief summary of your findings.
4. The file NY_Newborns.jmp contains information on newborn hospitalizations in New York State in 2016. Using this data, create a dashboard that can be used to explore variation in total cost of the hospitalizations. (Note that the total cost refers to the actual cost of a newborn's hospitalization, while the total charges are the amounts charged to insurers.)

4.9.5 Discussion Questions

1. Discuss the advantages of using a dashboard compared to the traditional paper report or a spreadsheet. Are there circumstances where a traditional report or spreadsheet might be a better option?
2. What are some ways to ensure that people using the dashboards are gaining insights from the visualizations provided in the dashboards?

References

Eckerson, W.W. (2011). *Performance Dashboards: Measuring, Monitoring, and Managing Your Business*, 2e. Wiley.

Hoerl, R. and Snee, R. (2012). *Statistical Thinking: Improving Business Performance*, 2e. Wiley.

JMP (2019). Dashboard building with JMP. https://www.jmp.com/en_us/ applications/dashboard-building.html (accessed 28 December 2019).

5

Variability in the Cost of Hip Replacement

5.1 Key Concepts

Variation, Data visualization, Descriptive statistics.

5.2 DMAIC

DMA: In this case, you will use tools that apply to the Define, Measure, and Analyze phases of the Define–Measure–Analyze–Improve–Control (DMAIC) process.

5.3 PDCA

PC: In this case, you will use tools that apply to the Plan and Check steps in the Plan–Do–Check–Act (PDCA) process.

5.4 Background

As healthcare costs continue to rise, consumers are actively seeking providers that deliver low cost, high-quality care. At the same time, the incidence of hip replacement (arthroplasty) surgery is increasing due to the aging "baby boomer" generation and younger people wishing to maintain an active lifestyle. High variability in the cost of hip replacement surgery has been reported in "A Study of Cost Variations in Knee and Hip Replacement Surgeries in the U.S." (Blue Cross Blue Shield 2015) and by the American Medical Association in "Availability of Consumer Prices from US Hospitals for a Common Surgical Procedure" (Rosenthal and Cram 2013).

Improving Health Care Quality: Case Studies with JMP®, First Edition.
Mary Ann Shifflet, Cecilia Martinez, Jane Oppenlander, and Shirley Shmerling.
© 2020 John Wiley & Sons, Inc. Published 2020 by John Wiley & Sons, Inc.
Books Companion site:www.wiley.com/go/shifflet/improvinghealthcarequality1e

The director of quality at an Upstate New York hospital is exploring possibilities for improving the hip replacement surgery process. To start, he would like to quantify the variability in the cost of hip replacement surgery at other regional hospitals. The New York State Department of Health makes in-patient hospital discharge data publicly available. This data will facilitate an initial understanding of the variability in the cost of hip replacement surgery at hospitals in the corresponding health service area. A health service area is a geographic subdivision of the State of New York. The Southern Tier is the region of New York State west of the Catskills that borders northern Pennsylvania.

5.5 The Task

In this case, we will examine the variability of the cost of hip replacement surgeries at hospitals in the Southern Tier of New York State.

5.6 The Data: SouthernTier_HipReplacement.csv

The Statewide Planning and Research Cooperative System (SPARCS) contains patient-level data collected by New York State for the purpose of providing healthcare organizations with information that will enable them to efficiently and cost effectively deliver services. This reporting system was established in 1979 and collects data on patient characteristics, diagnoses, treatments, and services for inpatient, ambulatory surgery, emergency department admission, and outpatient visits. The full data set contains personally identifiable information and as such, access is carefully controlled. However, a de-identified subset of the inpatient discharge data is made available to the public. We will use this de-identified data from 2016 to examine the total cost associated with hip replacement surgeries. SPARCS provides a web interface that allows subsets of the data to be downloaded in a variety of formats. The file SouthernTier_HipReplacement.csv was downloaded directly from SPARCS and contains information on hip replacement surgeries performed in hospitals in the Southern Tier Health Service Area. The data dictionary that gives the definition of each variable is provided with the data files that accompany this casebook. Total costs are defined as the actual cost of the services provided. Total charges are the amounts charged to insurers.

5.7 Data Management

The first step is to import the .csv file into JMP® and then prepare the data set for analysis. To import the .csv file into JMP, select **File > Open** and browse to the

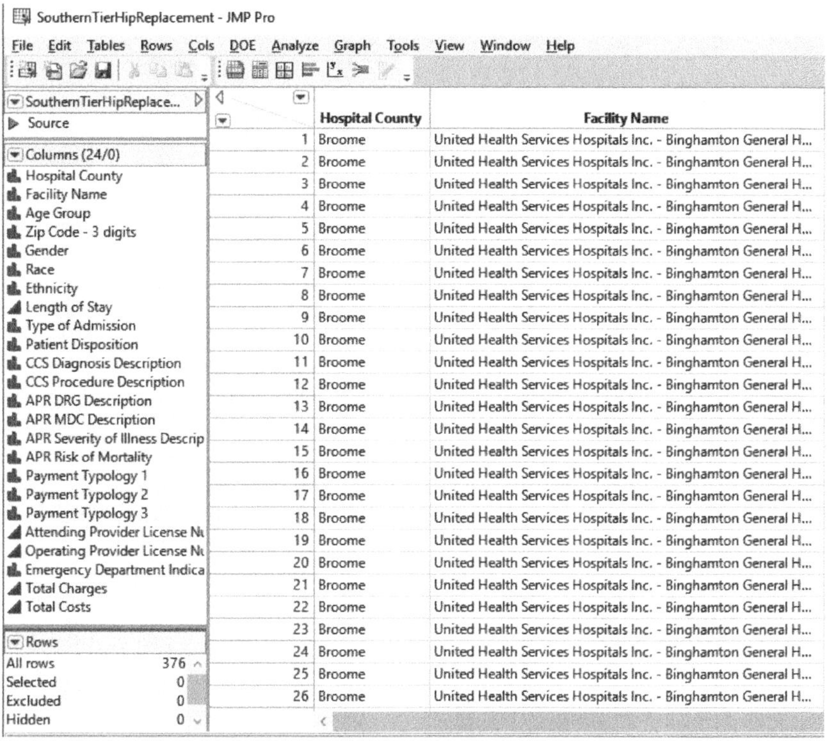

Figure 5.1 Data table column list.

location of SouthernTier_HipReplacement.csv. Figure 5.1 shows a portion of the JMP data table that includes the column list and the associated modeling type for each column.

5.7.1 Initial Data Review

JMP's Columns Viewer gives a simple overview of the variables in the data set. This is a good first step when examining new data to gain familiarity with it. Figure 5.2 shows the output for the Southern Tier hip replacement data.

In the Summary Statistics table, we see that there are 376 observations in this data set and the number of categories for columns imported as nominal variables are shown in **N Categories**. Facility Name has been imported as a nominal column with four categories. To see more detail for this column, highlight Facility Name, then click **Distribution**. The resulting output is shown in Figure 5.3.

For columns imported as a continuous variable, the minimum, maximum, mean, and standard deviation are shown. Based on the Columns Viewer output

Data Table Columns Viewer - JMP Pro — ☐ ✕

SouthernTierHipReplacement (376 rows, 37 columns)

▷ **Columns View Selector**

◢ ▼ **Summary Statistics**

37 Columns [Clear Select] [Distribution]

Columns	N	N Missing	N Categories	Min	Max	Mean	Std Dev
Health Service Area	376	0	1	.	.	.	.
Hospital County	376	0	2	.	.	.	.
Operating Certificate Number	376	0	.	301001	824000	366734.92021	170949.70282
Facility Id	376	0	.	42	128	54.311170213	27.999075846
Facility Name	376	0	4	.	.	.	.
Age Group	376	0	4	.	.	.	.
Zip Code - 3 digits	376	0	11	.	.	.	.
Gender	376	0	2	.	.	.	.
Race	376	0	3	.	.	.	.
Ethnicity	376	0	3	.	.	.	.
Length of Stay	376	0	.	1	26	3.2420212766	2.5123566965
Type of Admission	376	0	3	.	.	.	.
Patient Disposition	376	0	8	.	.	.	.
Discharge Year	376	0	.	2016	2016	2016	0
CCS Diagnosis Code	376	0	.	203	257	209.88829787	11.4560387
CCS Diagnosis Description	376	0	6	.	.	.	.
CCS Procedure Code	376	0	.	153	153	153	0
CCS Procedure Description	376	0	1	.	.	.	.
APR DRG Code	376	0	.	301	912	311.88031915	79.212383112
APR DRG Description	376	0	3	.	.	.	.
APR MDC Code	376	0	.	8	25	8.3005319149	2.1890880254
APR MDC Description	376	0	3	.	.	.	.
APR Severity of Illness Code	376	0	.	1	4	1.7845744681	0.7109627874
APR Severity of Illness Description	376	0	4	.	.	.	.
APR Risk of Mortality	376	0	4	.	.	.	.
APR Medical Surgical Description	376	0	1	.	.	.	.
Payment Typology 1	376	0	6	.	.	.	.
Payment Typology 2	288	88	5	.	.	.	.
Payment Typology 3	174	202	6	.	.	.	.
Attending Provider License Number	376	0	.	117067	90017719	444918.19149	4631822.7155
Operating Provider License Number	376	0	.	118213	285085	203898.86436	35514.981092
Other Provider License Number	0	376	0	.	.	.	.
Birth Weight	376	0	.	0	0	0	0
Abortion Edit Indicator	376	0	1	.	.	.	.
Emergency Department Indicator	376	0	2	.	.	.	.
Total Charges	376	0	.	1090.42	162130.35	44241.8825	16321.916421
Total Costs	376	0	.	4687.72	658260.4	15443.361223	5756.8929838

Figure 5.2 Columns viewer summary of hip replacement data.
(Cols > Column Viewer; Highlight all columns in the Select Columns field and click Show Summary.)

and domain knowledge, several data preparation steps are needed prior to analysis.

5.7.2 Adjusting JMP Column Properties

The modeling types assigned on import from the .csv file may not be appropriate and may need to be changed. For example, the Attending Provider License Number column was assigned a numeric modeling type; however, this is an identification number and should be treated as a nominal variable. To change the modeling type, right click the **modeling type icon** (blue triangle [gray in print] see Figure 5.1) and select **Nominal** from the dropdown menu. The modeling type icon will now appear as a red histogram (gray in print) in the column list in the JMP data table.

Some of the columns, such as All Patients Refined (APR) Risk of Mortality contain rating scale information. By default, JMP will present the levels in the

Distributions

Facility Name

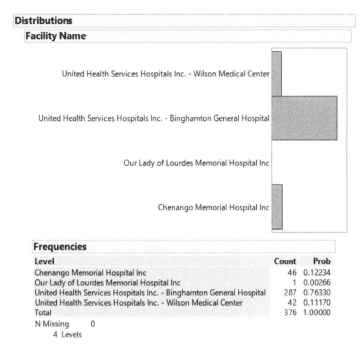

Frequencies

Level	Count	Prob
Chenango Memorial Hospital Inc	46	0.12234
Our Lady of Lourdes Memorial Hospital Inc	1	0.00266
United Health Services Hospitals Inc. - Binghamton General Hospital	287	0.76330
United Health Services Hospitals Inc. - Wilson Medical Center	42	0.11170
Total	376	1.00000

N Missing   0
    4 Levels

Figure 5.3 Distribution of Facility Name.

alphabetical order. This column should be changed to an ordinal modeling type and the Value Ordering column property applied so that levels are arranged in the appropriate order. Figure 5.4 shows the dialog used to set the order of the values.

5.7.3   Deleting Unneeded Columns

Deleting unneeded columns can reduce the size of the data table and simplify interactive analysis. However, the potential for growth in the scope of the analysis should be considered when choosing to delete columns. Several of the nominal columns, such as Health Service Area, contain only one category, and hence have no variability and are candidates for deletion. The scope of the current investigation is only the Southern Tier health service area, so this column could be deleted. However, if at a later date, other Health Service Areas may be analyzed, this column should be retained. Other columns, such as **Discharge Year** would be treated similarly.

The column Birth Weight contains only a single value of 0 for all observations. Birth weight is only recorded for newborns. This information is obtained from the SPARCS data dictionary, which is included with the files that accompany this casebook. This column does not contain useful information applicable to hip replacement and can be deleted. Abortion Edit Indicator can be treated similarly.

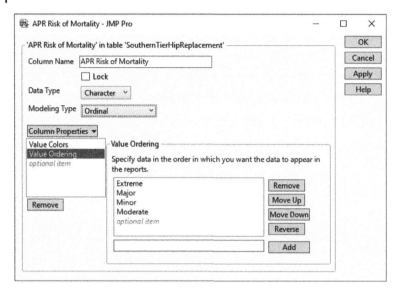

Figure 5.4 Setting value ordering for APR Risk of Mortality.
(Right click in the column header for APR Risk of Mortality; select Column Information. Select Ordinal from the Modeling Type dropdown menu. Select Value Ordering from the Column Properties dropdown and use the Move Up and Move Down buttons to reorder the values. Click Apply, then OK.)

SPARCS gives information on patient condition both as a description and as a numeric code, for example CCS (Clinical Classifications Software) Diagnosis Code and CCS Diagnosis Description. The decision to delete one of the columns with redundant information depends on the intended audience for communicating analytic results. Subject matter experts familiar with the codes may prefer their brevity while the descriptions may be more meaningful for other stakeholders.

The **Columns Viewer** output for **Other Provider License Number** shows that values for this column are missing for all 376 observations, so this column can be deleted from the data table. For this case study, a number of columns will be deleted, including those that contain numeric codes. Which columns to delete for any particular problem should balance the desire to reduce the size of the data table for ease of use and future needs to augment the analysis.

5.7.4 Shortening Character Columns

From Figure 5.3, we see that the Facility Name contains the full hospital name, which is lengthy and occupies a substantial amount of space on data visualizations. A new column can be created to hold the shortened facility names

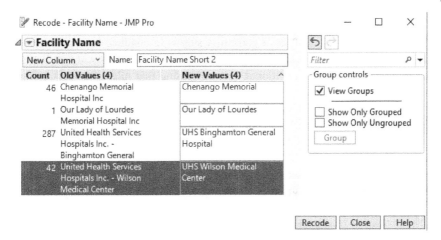

Figure 5.5 Recode dialog to create column for shortened Facility Name. (Cols > Recode. Edit text under New Values. Select New Column from the Done dropdown menu.)

using the JMP Recode feature. Figure 5.5 shows the completed **Recode** dialog. The **New Column** option has been selected.

The data is now ready for analysis and has been saved in the file Southern-Tier_HipReplacement.jmp.

5.8 Analysis

Statistical thinking is a philosophy, important in the quality culture, which recognizes that variation exists in all processes. Work in an organization is accomplished through interconnected systems of such processes. Successful process improvement is achieved by understanding and reducing variation in these systems.

It is expected that there is variation in patient medical conditions that contributes to the cost of hip replacement surgery. For example, an elderly patient or one with comorbidities may require longer lengths of stay or additional treatment that will result in higher cost. Such variation is largely outside of the control of the hospital. However, there may be variation due to hospital practices and procedures that could be reduced. Reducing variation can lead to increased efficiency and better use of resources, for example reduced wait times and fewer rescheduled appointments. In addition to improving the process of hip replacement from the hospital's perspective, patient satisfaction may increase with certain improvements such as reduced length of stay. An important part of the Analyze step of the DMAIC process is to understand the sources of process variability. We will focus on total cost to illustrate numerical and graphical methods for assessing variation.

5.8.1 Descriptive Analysis

At the start of a new analysis, a good first step is to conduct descriptive analysis of all pertinent variables in the data set, individually. This will familiarize you with the data, reveal additional data processing that might be needed, and provide insights for further analysis. Nominal and ordinal variables are summarized with frequency and relative frequency distributions; continuous variables are summarized using measures of centrality (mean and/or median) and measures of variation (standard deviation and/or interquartile range). Including the minimum and maximum provides the range of observed values. Figure 5.6 shows basic descriptive statistics for hospital geographic characteristics. Other variables can be described similarly and grouped into categories, such as patient demographics, discharge and payment, and patient medical condition.

In the hospital characteristics table (Figure 5.6), only the first three digits of the zip code are given. This is a technique used to de-identify patient-level data and protect privacy. The first three digits of the zip code identify the postal facility that

Tabulate

Hospital County	N	% of Total
Broome	330	87.8%
Chenango	46	12.2%
Facility Name Short		
Chenango Memorial	46	12.2%
Our Lady of Lourdes	1	0.3%
UHS Binghamton General Hospital	287	76.3%
UHS Wilson Medical Center	42	11.2%
Zip Code - 3 digits		
121	1	0.3%
124	1	0.3%
130	1	0.3%
131	1	0.3%
133	1	0.3%
134	3	0.8%
137	129	34.3%
138	115	30.6%
139	99	26.3%
148	5	1.3%
OOS	20	5.3%

Figure 5.6 Descriptive statistics for hospital geographic characteristics. (Analyze > Tabulate. Drag column names to Row Drop Zone, drag statistics to Column Drop Zone. Check Include missing for grouping columns. Click Set Format and adjust rounding.)

Tabulate

Type of Admission	N	% of Total
Elective	299	79.5%
Emergency	76	20.2%
Urgent	1	0.3%
Emergency Department Indicator		
N	307	81.6%
Y	69	18.4%

Figure 5.7 Descriptive statistics for patient admission.

is the center for mail sorting and distribution in a geographic area (USPS n.d.). Another de-identification method employed in the SPARCS data is to aggregate values such as age that could be used to identify an individual.

Figure 5.7 shows the descriptive statistics for the variables associated with patient admission. There is an apparent discrepancy between the two variables where Type of Admission shows 76 emergency admissions, while the Emergency Department Indicator variables show 69. The data dictionary indicates that these two variables are defined differently, and this is why the frequencies are not the same. The Emergency Department Indicator variables is defined as "The Emergency Department Indicator is set based on the submitted revenue codes. If the record contained an Emergency Department revenue code of 045X, the indicator is set to 'Y,' otherwise, it will be 'N.'" (New York State Department of Health, 2019). A best practice is to carefully review the variable definitions found in the data dictionary that accompanies a data set.

5.8.2 Assessing Variability

Data visualizations are a good way to begin assessing variability. Since the cost of hip replacement is of interest, a histogram showing the distribution of total cost is given in Figure 5.8.

The histogram shows that most of the costs lie between $10,000 and $20,000, the distribution has a slight right skew, and there is a large outlier where the cost is close to $70,000. The outlier box plot above the histogram is a more compact way to show the distribution. The box defines the interquartile range (25th percentile to 75th percentile), the vertical line inside the box is the median, the diamond indicates the mean and its 95% confidence interval, and the bracket above the box shows the densest 50% of the data. The whiskers are defined as 1.5 times the interquartile range (75th percentile to 25th percentile) below the first quartile and 1.5 times the interquartile range above the third quartile. Observations beyond the whiskers are considered outliers and appear as dots on the box plot.

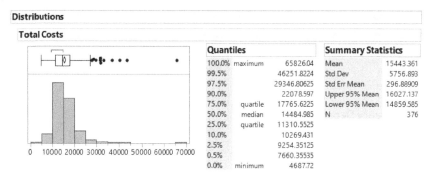

Figure 5.8 Distribution output for total cost. (Analyze > Distribution.)

To highlight the most extreme outlier in the data table, click on the data dot in the box plot. When investigating this observation in the data table we see that the patient is a white male, 70 years or older who was admitted through the emergency department of the Wilson Medical Center. The unusually high cost was likely due to a 26-day length of stay, severity of illness rated as major, and a moderate risk of mortality. While the total cost is comparatively high for this patient, it appears consistent with the available information on the patient's age and health status; there is no reason to remove this observation from the data set.

The histogram reveals that there is considerable variability in the cost of hip replacements in the Southern Tier; the standard deviation is $5,757 and the range (maximum–minimum) is $61,139. This variability is consistent with what was reported by Blue Cross Blue Shield (2015) and Rosenthal and Cram (2013).

In deciding if the hip replacement surgery process is a candidate for a process improvement project, assessing the variability in each Southern Tier hospital may provide insight. In Figure 5.6, we saw that Our Lady of Lourdes Hospital only reported one hip replacement in 2016. It is not possible to assess variability with only one observation, so before conducting further analysis, the data table should be modified to exclude the single observation associated with this hospital. Since we are looking for one record to exclude, JMP's search function can locate the record. Figure 5.9 shows the completed dialog.

To create histograms of total cost for each hospital in one display, use JMP's Graph Builder as shown in Figure 5.10. Notice that the histograms are plotted on the same axis scale so that they can be compared. The distributions for all three hospitals are quite similar, and all are slightly right skewed. Binghamton General Hospital performs many more hip replacement surgeries than the other two hospitals.

Figure 5.11 shows an alternative visualization of the variability by hospital using box plots. The box plots allow outliers to be easily identified and the center and variation of the hospital cost distribution to be compared.

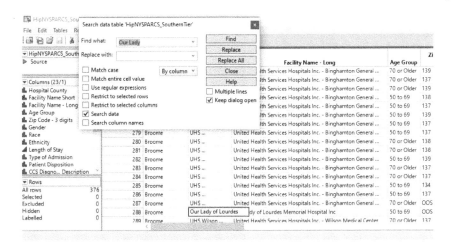

Figure 5.9 Search dialog to find Our Lady of Lourdes Hospital observation.
(Edit > Search. Complete dialog as shown. Click Find. Right click the row where Our Lady of Lourdes is identified and select Hide and Exclude.)

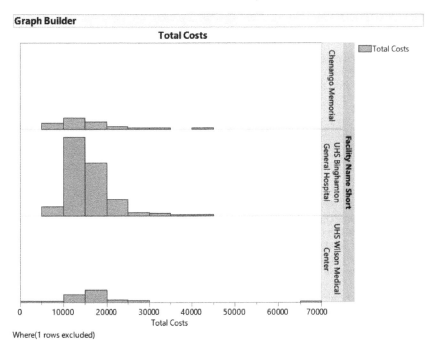

Figure 5.10 Total cost histograms by hospital.
(Graph > Graph Builder. Drag Total Cost into the X drop zone. Drag Facility Name Short into the Y drop zone. Select the histogram icon from the Control Panel.)

Graph Builder

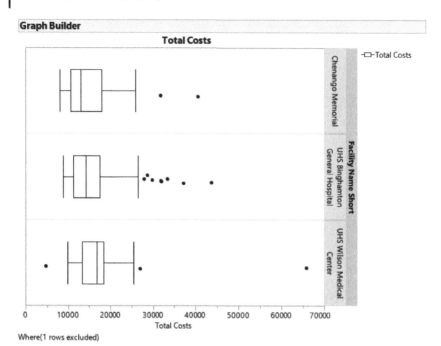

Where(1 rows excluded)

Figure 5.11 Total cost box plots by hospital.
(Graph > Graph Builder. Drag Total Cost into the X drop zone. Drag Facility Name Short into the Group Y drop zone. Select the Box Plot icon from the Control Panel.)

Tabulate

	Facility Name Short	N	% of Total	Mean	Median	Std Dev	Min	Max	Range
Total Costs	Chenango Memorial	46	11.9%	15025	12980	6421	8047	40556	32509
	UHS Binghamton General Hospital	287	75.4%	15198	14244	5038	8763	43708	34945
	UHS Wilson Medical Center	42	12.7%	17499	16694	8693	4688	65826	61138

1 row has been excluded.

Figure 5.12 Descriptive statistics for cost by hospital.
(Analyze > Tabulate. Drag Total Cost to drop zone for rows; drag Facility Name Short to the column just to the right of Total Cost. Drag Sum to column header above the values. Highlight N, % of Total, Mean, Median, Std Dev, Min, Max, and Range and drag over top of Sum in the column header. Click Change Format and adjust the number of digits displayed to show only whole dollars.)

Figure 5.12 shows a table of descriptive statistics for total costs by hospital. Notice that the output shows that one observation has been excluded from the analysis. Recall that this is the observation from Our Lady of Lourdes Hospital.

Comparing the centrality measures, we see that the means are quite similar for Chenango Memorial and Binghamton General Hospitals, with Wilson Medical Center having a larger mean, likely influenced by the large outlier observed in the box plot. The medians are within a few thousand dollars of each other. The variation measures (standard deviation and range) are likewise similar for Chenango Memorial and Binghamton General Hospitals.

5.9 Summary

5.9.1 Statistical Insights

In this case, we have seen that considerable effort was needed to prepare a downloaded data file for analysis. An initial descriptive analysis can identify data anomalies (e.g. missing data) and familiarize the analyst with the data. An apparent contradiction in the two variables that deal with emergency department admissions was resolved by consulting the data dictionary where a subtle difference in definitions was discovered. In preparing a data set for analysis, the desire to work with a smaller data table, achieved by deleting variables that seem not to be pertinent, or have no variability, must be balanced with anticipated future analysis and problem scope changes.

Data visualizations and tables of numerical statistics are useful to assess variability. A best practice is to begin with univariate descriptive analysis, proceed to bivariate analysis, and then multivariate analysis. Examining histograms and tables of descriptive statistics revealed considerable variability in the total cost of hip replacement, consistent with reported findings. The patterns of variability for the three hospitals in the Southern Tier were similar. Binghamton General Hospital performed 75% of all hip replacements in the Southern Tier in 2016. It could be hypothesized that this volume would be associated with lower costs due to economies of scale; however, this was not apparent in the analysis.

5.9.2 Implications and Next Steps

The purpose of this analysis was to help inform a decision on whether to pursue a quality improvement project in the hip replacement surgery process. The results showed variability in total cost in this region by hospital that is consistent with high variability reported nationally. The hip replacement surgery process, due to its high cost variability, provides an opportunity for quality improvement, and its selection would depend on resources available for this project and other possible projects under consideration.

While this descriptive analysis revealed no marked differences in the variability between hospitals with respect to total cost, there may be other variables to consider. For example, a regional medical center may receive more difficult cases than a community hospital. In the Measure and Analyze phases of the DMAIC cycle, additional analysis should be conducted to identify and quantify the sources of variability and determine those that are under the hospital's control (e.g. preoperative, operative, and postoperative processes) and those that are not under the hospital's control (e.g. underlying patient medical condition and comorbidities.)

Further research should be conducted to identify other hospitals outside of the region that have lower and less variable total costs for hip replacement surgery or those that have conducted quality improvement projects for this process. Such benchmarking can further inform the decision whether to further pursue the hip replacement surgery process for a quality improvement initiative.

5.9.3 Summary of Tools and JMP Features

Statistical methods tools	Data management tasks concepts	JMP platform features	Quality tools
Data visualization	Data cleansing	Column viewer	Process variation
– *Histogram*			
– *Box plot*			
Descriptive statistics	De-identification	Distribution	Sources of variation
Outlier analysis		Column properties	Statistical thinking
		– *Modeling type*	
		– *Value ordering*	
		Recode	
		Tabulate	
		Edit > Search	
		Graph builder	

5.9.4 Exercises

1. Select the variables that should be in a table of descriptive statistics for payment and discharge characteristics. Use JMP's Tabulate feature to create a table of descriptive statistics for the chosen variables.
2. Prepare a descriptive analysis of patient demographics and medical condition by hospital using tables of numerical statistics and data visualizations. How is the information useful in understanding variations in total cost by hospital?

3. Examine the effect of the large outlier (total cost of $65,826) for Wilson Medical Center by creating a table of descriptive statistics similar to that of Figure 5.12 excluding the outlier. What is the influence of this observation on the centrality measures (mean and median) and the variation measures (standard deviation and range)?

4. Download the 2016 data from the NY Southern Tier Health Service Area for knee replacement surgery (search terms: SPARCS 2016 de-identified; CCS Procedure code 152) and assess the variation using the techniques illustrated in this case. Compare the variation in the total cost of knee replacement surgery to that of hip replacement surgery making note of differences and similarities.

5. Select a condition or procedure of interest to you and download the SPARCS data for a year and region of your choice (search terms: SPARCS de-identified).

   (a) Assess the variation in the total cost using the techniques illustrated in this case.

   (b) Search the Internet for published information on the cost of your chosen condition or procedure. Discuss how your results compare to what you found in your research.

   (c) Search the Internet for published quality improvements associated with your chosen condition/procedure. Do any of the improvements involve variables available in the SPARCS data?

   (d) Summarize your findings in a brief report.

5.9.5 Discussion Questions

1. What variables in the data set would you expect to influence the variability in total cost of hip replacement surgery? Create histograms and box plots using these variables, similar to Figures 5.10 and 5.11 to visualize the variability. Are the histograms consistent with your expectations? Why or why not?

2. A large percentage of knee and hip replacement surgeries are elective, which allows consumers time to evaluate the cost and quality associated with different surgeons and hospitals. This is not the case with procedures that are done on an emergency or urgent basis.

   (a) What other variables, not available in the SPARCS de-identified data, do you think consumers electing to have joint replacement surgery might consider when choosing a surgeon or hospital?

   (b) Look for published reports or studies that help corroborate the variables you identified in part (a).

   (c) Is data publicly available on these variables? If not, how would you recommend collecting this data?

References

Blue Cross Blue Shield (2015, January 21). A study of cost variations for knee and hip replacement surgeries in the U.S. Retrieved from https://www.bcbs.com/the-health-of-america/reports/study-of-cost-variations-knee-and-hip-replacement-surgeries-the-us.

New York State Department of Health, Office of Quality and Patient Safety. (2019, September). Hospital Inpatient Discharges (SPARCS De-Identified File) DATA DICTIONARY. Retrieved from https://health.data.ny.gov/w/tsg2-5hds/fbc6-cypp?cur=9H1SBRZOtZ0&from=root.

Rosenthal, X., Lu, J.A., and Cram, P. (2013). Availability of consumer prices from us hospitals for a common surgical procedure. *JAMA Internal Medicine* 173 (6): 424–432.

United States Postal Service. (n.d.). Definitions. Publication 220 - Discount "Postal Customer" Mailings: A Guide for the House of Representatives. Retrieved from https://about.usps.com/publications/pub220/pub220c2.htm.

6

Benchmarking the Cost of Hip Replacement

6.1 Key Concepts

Hypothesis testing, confidence intervals.

6.2 DMAIC

A: In this case you will use tools that apply to the Analyze phase in the Define–Measure–Analyze–Improve–Control (DMAIC) process.

6.3 PDCA

DC: In this case, you will use tools that apply to the Do and Check steps in the Plan–Do–Check–Act (PDCA) process.

6.4 Background

In the case "Variability in the Cost of Hip Replacement" (Chapter 5), we quantified the variability of the cost of hip replacement in the Southern Tier region of New York, both graphically and numerically. We found this region to have high variability in hip replacement cost, consistent with what has been reported nationally (Blue Cross Blue Shield, 2015; Rosenthal and Cram, 2013).

In continuous improvement, benchmarking is a valuable tool to compare current performance with other institutions. Hospitals can compare their performance with regional competitors or those that are best-in-class nationally or

Improving Health Care Quality: Case Studies with JMP®, First Edition.
Mary Ann Shifflet, Cecilia Martinez, Jane Oppenlander, and Shirley Shmerling.
© 2020 John Wiley & Sons, Inc. Published 2020 by John Wiley & Sons, Inc.
Books Companion site:www.wiley.com/go/shifflet/improvinghealthcarequality1e

internationally. Benchmarking opportunities can involve the exchange of data or best practices between organizations, on-site visits to observe and discuss operations and processes, or the use of published reports and rankings. Benchmarking can identify opportunities for improvement and guide the selection of improvement initiatives.

In this case, we will benchmark the cost of hip replacement for one of the Southern Tier hospitals against a best-in-class market as reported by Blue Cross Blue Shield in "The Health of America Report: A Study of Cost Variations for Knee and Hip Replacement Surgeries in the U.S." Blue Cross Blue Shield (2015).

6.5 The Task

This case compares mean cost of hip replacement at the United Health Services Hospitals Wilson Medical Center in the Southern Tier of New York to that of the best-in-class hospitals using a statistical test of hypothesis. In addition, we will find an 95% confidence interval for the mean cost of hip replacement for the Wilson Medical Center.

6.6 The Data: HipNYSPARCS_SouthernTier.jmp

We return to the data from "Variability in the Cost of Hip Replacement" in Chapter 5 and select a subset of that data for use in this case. The data source is New York State's Statewide Planning and Research Cooperative System (SPARCS) which provides healthcare organizations with patient-level data to enable them to efficiently and cost effectively deliver services. This reporting system was established in 1979 and collects data on patient characteristics, diagnoses, treatments, and services for inpatient, ambulatory surgery, emergency department admission, and outpatient visits. The full data set contains personally identifiable information and access is carefully controlled. A subset of the inpatient discharge data is made available to the public. We will use the 2016 de-identified data for total cost of hospitalization for hip replacement surgery. Total costs are the actual costs of the services provided. Data definitions can be found in the downloadable data dictionary (New York State Department of Health 2016) which is provided with the data files that accompany this casebook.

6.7 Data Management

The data downloaded from the SPARCS website was prepared for analysis in Chapter 5 and contains the data from all hospitals in the Southern Tier health service area. For this case, only the data from the Wilson Medical Center is needed.

JMP'®s Data Filter is an easy way to select a subset of data. To create a subset containing only the Wilson Medical Center data, select Rows > Data Filter. Highlight Facility Name Short in the Add Filter Columns field and click the Add button. Highlight UHS – Wilson Medical Center and the rows corresponding to this hospital will be selected. Return to the data table and select Tables > Subset, then click OK in the resulting dialog. A new data table appears with only the rows for the Wilson Medical Center. Save the data table as a file by selecting File > Save as and enter Wilson_HipReplacement.jmp. Close the Data Filter.

6.8 Analysis

6.8.1 Descriptive Analysis

Always begin an analysis by familiarizing yourself with the data using descriptive statistics and data visualizations. Figure 6.1 shows the Distribution output for Total Cost.

The key centrality measures are the mean of $17,499 and the median of $16,694. The mean is sensitive to the large outlier that can be seen in the histogram and the box plot; the median, which is based on only the middle observation(s), is not sensitive to the outlier, and thus is smaller than the mean. The standard deviation of $8,693 is a measure of variation. The minimum of $4,688 and the maximum of $65,826 provide the range of the observed total costs.

6.8.2 Statistical Test of Hypothesis

Blue Cross Blue Shield (2015) identified the US markets that reported the highest and lowest costs for both knee and hip replacement surgery. The best performing

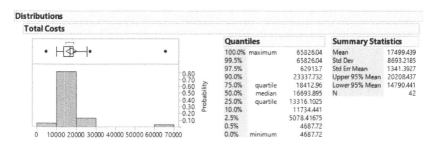

Figure 6.1 Summary Statistics for total cost of hip replacement for Wilson Medical Center.
(Analyze > Distribution; Drag Total Cost to Y, Column.)

market for hip replacement was Montgomery, Alabama, with the lowest average cost of approximately $16,500. We will compare the average total cost for the Wilson Medical Center with this benchmark.

From Figure 6.1, we see that the mean total cost for Wilson Medical Center is $17,499, which is larger than the best-in-class value of $16,500. To see if the difference is significant, a statistical test of hypothesis is performed. The purpose of a hypothesis test is to evaluate the difference in light of sampling error. Sampling error is the precision with which the mean total cost has been estimated. When comparing a single mean to a benchmark value, a one-sample t-test is an appropriate method. For additional detail on the one-sample t-test see Polit (2010) or Rosner (2015).

The first step in conducting a hypothesis test is to set up the null and alternative hypotheses. The null hypothesis assumes that the mean for Wilson Medical Center is equal to the benchmark of $16,500. The statistical notation used to represent this null hypothesis is H_0: $\mu = 16,500$. The alternative hypothesis can be specified in one of three ways, depending on the research question. A two-sided alternative (H_a: $\mu \neq 16,500$) tests if the mean for Wilson Medical Center differs from the benchmark. There are two possible one-sided alternative hypotheses, the mean is less than the benchmark or the mean is greater than the benchmark. A two-sided alternative hypothesis is the appropriate choice in this case since we are looking to see if the average cost of hip replacement for Wilson Medical Center is different from the benchmark.

Once the null and alternative hypotheses are specified, the hypothesis test can be conducted with the JMP Distribution platform. Figure 6.2 shows the output.

The p-value is the key result from a hypothesis test, and since it is a probability, it is defined on a scale between 0 and 1. Small p-values (typically less than 0.05) result in rejection of the null hypothesis (support for the alternative hypothesis) and large p-values result in not rejecting the null hypothesis (no support for

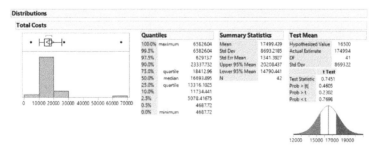

Figure 6.2 Test of hypotheses results for Wilson Medical Center Total Cost. (Analyze > Distribution. Select Test Mean from the dropdown menu (red arrow). Enter 16500 in the Specify Hypothesized Mean field. Click OK.)

the alternative hypothesis). The p-value is the likelihood of obtaining the sample mean or a value more extreme assuming the null hypothesis is true. The JMP Distribution output gives the p-values associated with each of the three possible alternative hypotheses. They appear as the three values at the bottom of the Test Mean table. The bell-shaped distribution below the three p-values illustrates how the p-value is determined. The bell is the sampling distribution of the mean, centered at the hypothesized value of $16,500 and scaled by the standard error of the mean ($1,341). The shaded areas in the tails show the p-value associated with the two-sided alternative. For our two-sided alternative, Prob $>|t| = 0.4605$, is the p-value. In this case, the null hypothesis is not rejected at the 5% significance level since the p-value of 0.4605 is not less than the significance level of 0.05. The difference of $999 between the mean total cost for Wilson Medical Center and the benchmark of $16,500 is not large enough to be considered statistically significant in light of the precision with which the mean for Wilson Medical Center was estimated. Therefore, we can conclude that Wilson Medical Center is performing, statistically, the same as the national best-in-class market with respect to cost. Additional information on hypothesis testing can be found in Rosner (2015) and Polit (2010).

6.8.3 Confidence Interval for Mean Total Cost

A confidence interval is computed from the sample data and gives a range of plausible values for the true parameter, in this case the mean total cost. Confidence intervals take the precision with which the mean was estimated into account. A 95% confidence interval for total cost is from $14,790 to $20,208, as shown in Figure 6.2 under the **Summary Statistics** portion of the **Distribution** output. There is 95% confidence that the true mean cost of hip replacement surgery for Wilson Medical Center lies between $14,790 and $20,208. Confidence intervals with other confidence levels (e.g. 90%, 99%) can be found by using the Confidence Interval option from the Total Cost dropdown menu. Additional explanation of confidence intervals can be found in Polit (2010) or Rosner (2015).

6.9 Summary

6.9.1 Statistical Insights

In the context of managing quality, simply comparing a mean calculated from data to a benchmark value is not sufficient. Statistical significance is established by testing hypotheses with the p-value being the key result. While the difference of $999 between Wilson Medical Center and the benchmark value appears to be a substantial savings, it was found to be statistically insignificant. Allocating resources to make process changes should be based, at least in part, on establishing statistical significance.

6.9.2 Implications and Next Steps

The results of the statistical hypothesis test show that Wilson Medical Center's mean cost is not statistically different from the cost of a national best-in-class benchmark. The large outlier warrants further investigation (see Exercise 2).

There are many other factors to consider that could warrant process improvement efforts. For example, patient outcomes, or procedural, regulatory or policy differences. In this case, we have illustrated how statistical tests of hypothesis and confidence intervals are valuable tools that can help in allocating resources wisely for process improvements.

6.9.3 Summary of Tools and JMP Features

Statistical methods tools	Data management concepts	JMP platform features	Quality tools
Descriptive statistics	Subsetting	Data filter	Benchmarking
Data visualization		Tables > Subset	
– *Histogram*			
Hypothesis test for a mean			
Confidence interval for a mean			

6.9.4 Exercises

1. Conduct a statistical test of hypothesis to determine if the mean total cost of hip replacement at UHS Binghamton General Hospital is different from $16,500.
   (a) Create a table of descriptive statistics for Total Cost using Tabulate.
   (b) Set up the appropriate null and alternative hypotheses.
   (c) Conduct the hypothesis test and state the result.
   (d) Find a 95% confidence interval for the mean total cost for hip replacement at UHS Binghamton General Hospital. Give an interpretation of the confidence interval.
   (e) Explain how a statistical test of hypothesis differs from a confidence interval and when to use each.

(f) Compare the results from UHS Binghamton General Hospital to those of Wilson Medical Center. Discuss reasons for similarities and differences you observe.

2. Repeat the statistical hypothesis test and confidence interval calculation performed in this case with the large outlier excluded. Describe how this outlier affects the hypothesis test and the confidence interval. Do your conclusions differ from those using all of the data? If the conclusions differ, what is your recommendation for handling the outlier?

3. Compute a 95% confidence interval for the standard deviation of the cost of hip replacement hospitalization at Wilson Medical Center. Give an interpretation of this interval.

4. Download the 2016 data from the NY Southern Tier Health Service Area for knee replacement surgery (CCS Procedure code 152). Conduct a statistical test of hypothesis to determine if the mean cost for the Southern Tier differs from that of the best performing market (Montgomery, Alabama) which reported an average cost of $16,100.

5. Select a condition or procedure of interest to you and download the SPARCS data for a year and region of your choice.

(a) Search the Internet for published information on the cost of your chosen condition or procedure. Find a cost value to use as a benchmark. Explain why you chose the benchmark you did.

(b) Prepare a descriptive analysis for your data using appropriate visualizations and tables of numerical statistics.

(c) Conduct a test of hypothesis that compares the mean cost of your chosen procedure/condition to the benchmark value you obtained.

(d) Discuss what the results of your hypothesis test mean in the context of process improvements to achieve cost reduction.

6. What are the assumptions that underlie a hypothesis test for a single mean? (*Hint*: Consult an outside reference.) Does the data used in this case satisfy these assumptions? If not, what alternative methods can be used?

6.9.5 Discussion Questions

1. Research sources that can be used to obtain benchmarking values for various healthcare quality indicators (e.g. hospital acquired conditions). Discuss your findings and how they might be used in process improvement efforts.

2. Search the literature to find reports or articles that use hypothesis testing in process improvement. Summarize the article in a few paragraphs and explain how the hypothesis tests were used to achieve process improvement.

3. Research the concept of practical (or clinical) significance and compare it to statistical significance. Discuss how each of these concepts can be applied in process improvement.

References

Blue Cross Blue Shield (2015, January 21). A study of cost variations for knee and hip replacement surgeries in the U.S. Retrieved from https://www.bcbs.com/the-health-of-america/reports/study-of-cost-variations-knee-and-hip-replacement-surgeries-the-us.

New York State Department of Health (2016). Hospital inpatient discharges (SPARCS de-identified): 2016. *Health Data NY*. Retrieved from https://health.data.ny.gov/Health/Hospital-Inpatient-Discharges-SPARCS-De-Identified/gnzp-ekau.

Polit, D.F. (2010). *Statistics and Data Analysis for Nursing Research*, 2e). Pearson.

Rosenthal, X., Lu, J.A., and Cram, P. (2013). Availability of consumer prices from us hospitals for a common surgical procedure. *JAMA Internal Medicine* 173 (6): 424–432.

Rosner, B. (2015). *Fundamentals of Biostatistics*, 8e. Cengage Learning.

7

Nursing Survey

7.1 Key Concepts

Descriptive statistics, data visualization, tests of hypothesis for proportions, confidence intervals for proportions.

7.2 DMAIC

A: The tools illustrated in this case are frequently applied in the Analyze phase of the Define–Measure–Analyze–Improve–Control (DMAIC) approach to process improvement.

7.3 PDCA

DC: In this case, you will use tools that apply to the Do and Check steps in the Plan–Do–Check–Act (PDCA) process.

7.4 Background

A 450-bed general acute care hospital is pursuing "magnet" designation, which is awarded by the American Nurses Credentialing Center for demonstrated excellence in nursing. A number of benefits accrue to magnet hospitals, including high-quality patient care, high levels of job satisfaction among the nursing staff, and the ability to attract and retain high-quality nursing staff. Achieving magnet

Improving Health Care Quality: Case Studies with JMP®, First Edition.
Mary Ann Shifflet, Cecilia Martinez, Jane Oppenlander, and Shirley Shmerling.
© 2020 John Wiley & Sons, Inc. Published 2020 by John Wiley & Sons, Inc.
Books Companion site:www.wiley.com/go/shifflet/improvinghealthcarequality1e

designation requires hospitals to demonstrate excellence in five areas, one of which is evidence-based practice (EBP), which is an approach to patient care that integrates nursing research, a nurse's clinical experience and skill, and patient values.

One area of concern is the adequacy of the nursing research holdings in the medical library. To assess the situation, the Nursing Research and Evidence-based Practice Council is benchmarking with other similarly sized hospitals in the region and utilizing the results of a survey given to the hospital's registered nurses to assess the nursing culture. The survey is a validated instrument (Gale and Schaffer, 2009) covering a number of areas related to EBP, including the adequacy of access to nursing literature.

Assessing the nurses' satisfaction with the adequacy of nursing literature is an example of obtaining the "voice of the customer." Both benchmarking and developing an understanding of the voice of the customer are best practices in quality improvement.

7.5   The Task

The objective of this case is to assess the nursing survey questions related to the availability of nursing literature to gauge the nurses' satisfaction with the hospital's resources. It was also of interest to the Nursing Research and Evidence-based Practice Council to know if the perceptions differed between staff nurses and those in nursing leadership positions.

7.6   The Data: NursingResearch_Survey_Responses.jmp

The survey was reviewed and approved by the hospital's Institutional Review Board (IRB). US federal law requires organizations conducting biomedical or behavioral research to have an IRB that evaluates research studies to ensure the protection of human subjects. The survey was then offered to all 854 registered nurses employed by the hospital. The first survey question asked respondents to give their consent to participate. If consent was not given, the survey application closed. Of the nurses who accessed the survey, 262 (30.7%) agreed to participate.

The data from the seven survey questions and respondent demographics are contained in the file NursingResearch_Survey_Responses.jmp. The survey questions asked each respondent to rate each proposition on a 5-point Likert agreement scale. The survey questions and definitions of the other variables collected are shown in Table 7.1.

Table 7.1 Data definitions for nursing survey responses.

Do you agree to participate in this survey?	Yes/no
Application of evidence-based practice is essential for effective nursing practice	Strongly disagree/disagree/neutral/agree/strongly agree
Literature and research findings are useful in my daily practice	Strongly disagree/disagree/neutral/agree/strongly agree
The adoption of evidence-based practice puts an unreasonable demand on my time	Strongly disagree/disagree/neutral/agree/strongly agree
Evidence-based practice does not take into account the limitations of my practice setting	Strongly disagree/disagree/neutral/agree/strongly agree
Evidence-based practice helps me make decisions about patient care	Strongly disagree/disagree/neutral/agree/strongly agree
There is sufficient information available for me to access when I have questions about the practice change	Strongly disagree/disagree/neutral/agree/strongly agree
All of the practice changes so far have been practical and fit well with the workflow of the unit	Strongly disagree/disagree/neutral/agree/strongly agree
Primary role	Job title – nurse manager, associate nurse manager, nurse educator/quality specialist or registered nurse
Year of service	Number of years employed as a nurse in this hospital
Employment status	Full-time, part-time, or per diem
Education	Highest nursing degree held

7.7 Data Management

Several data process steps must be completed to prepare the file for analysis.

7.7.1 Initial Data Review

The JMP® Columns Viewer is a convenient way to do an initial review of the data to discover anomalies such as missing data and columns that should be assigned a different JMP modeling type. Figure 7.1 shows the Columns Viewer output for the survey responses.

JMP has assigned all columns in this data table a nominal modeling type. The rating questions are, however, measured on a Likert scale, which is an ordinal

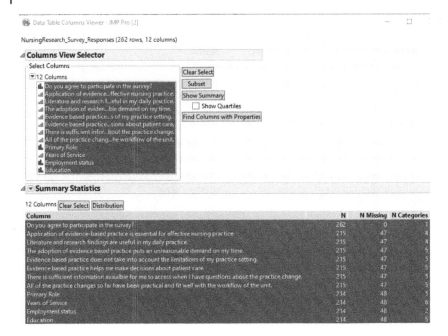

Figure 7.1 Columns Viewer output for survey responses.
(Cols > Columns Viewer. Select all columns in the Select Columns field. Click Show
Summary.)

scale. The modeling type should be changed to Ordinal for the Likert scale
questions by right-clicking the icon to the left of the column name in the Select
Columns field (see Figure 7.1) and select Ordinal from the dropdown menu.

From this output, we see that the first column corresponds to the consent question, the next seven columns are the rating questions, and the last four columns
are the demographic questions. An interesting pattern of missing data can be seen
in the N Missing column where there are 47 missing observations for the rating
questions and 48 missing observations for the demographic variables. Creating
a Missing Data Pattern table will give additional detail. A portion of the table is
shown in Figure 7.2.

This table gives the frequency and number of columns missing for each missing data pattern. The Patterns column contains a coded string representing the
columns analyzed, with a 0 indicating that there are no missing values in a column and a 1 indicating that there are missing values in that column. For example,
there are 214 rows that have complete information (a pattern of all zeros). There is
one instance where the last four columns have missing values. This corresponds to
the four demographic columns. There are 47 columns where all columns contain
missing values except for the consent question. This indicates that once the survey

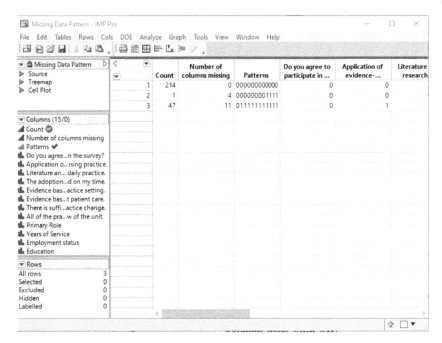

Figure 7.2 Missing Data Pattern table for survey responses.
(Tables > Missing Data Pattern. Select all columns in the Add Columns field. Click OK.)

application was opened, 47 respondents either chose not to provide any information or there were technical problems that prevented these responses from being saved. Since these 47 rows do not contain any meaningful information, they can be removed from the data table. This can be accomplished by selecting row 3 in the Missing Data Pattern table. Notice when that row is selected the 47 rows in the original data set are also highlighted. If you go back to the original data table, you can then delete those 47 rows that have been selected. Save the data table with File > Save.

7.7.2 Recoding the Primary Role Column

One of the objectives of this analysis is to determine if there are differences in how staff nurses perceive the availability of nursing literature as compared to nurse leaders. However, there is not a column that indicates whether a respondent is in a leadership position. This information can be derived from a respondent's job title, which is given in the Primary Role column. The hospital defines a nurse leader as either a nurse manager, an associate nurse manager, or a nurse educator/quality specialist. A new column containing the organizational level for each respondent can be created with JMP's Recode feature as shown in Figure 7.3.

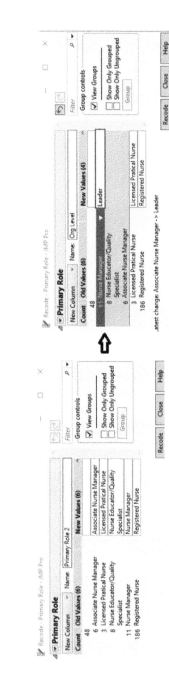

Figure 7.3 Recoding the Primary Role column.
(Cols > Recode. Select Primary Role. In Name field type Org Level. Type new values into New Values, column. Click Recode.)

Note that there are three respondents with a primary role of Licensed Practical Nurse as can be seen in the Old Values column. Only registered nurses were eligible to take this survey, therefore, these three responses should be removed. The data table is now ready for analysis and has been saved as NursingResearch_Survey_Responses_processed.jmp with a total of 212 responses. This gives a response rate of 24.8% for this survey.

7.8 Analysis

The survey question, "There is sufficient information available for me to access when I have questions about the practice change" will address the analysis objective, and thus, will be the focus of this case.

7.8.1 Descriptive Analysis

Always begin an analysis by familiarizing yourself with the key variables by using descriptive statistics and data visualizations. Figure 7.4 shows a statistical summary of the respondent demographics created with JMP Tabulate.

Figure 7.4 Nursing survey respondent demographics.
(Analyze > Tabulate. Drag Primary Role, Org Level, Years of Service, Employment status, and Education to the Drop zone for rows. Drag N and % of Total to the Drop zone for columns. Check Include missing for grouping columns. Select Change Format. In the % of Total field change the 2 to 1 to display percentages to one decimal place.)

Tabulate

Primary Role	N	% of Total
Missing	1	0.5%
Associate Nurse Manager	6	2.8%
Nurse Educator/Quality Specialist	8	3.8%
Nurse Manager	11	5.8%
Registered Nurse	186	87.7%
Org Level		
Missing	1	0.5%
Nurse Leader	25	11.8%
Staff Nurse	186	87.7%
Years of Service		
Missing	1	0.5%
Less than one year	20	9.4%
1 – 3 years	42	19.8%
3 – 5 years	32	15.1%
5 – 10 years	42	19.8%
10 – 20 years	28	13.2%
20 years +	47	22.2%
Employment status		
Missing	1	0.5%
Full Time	176	83.0%
Part Time/Per Diem	35	16.5%
Education		
Missing	1	0.5%
Associate's	126	59.4%
Bachelor's	52	24.5%
Diploma	20	9.4%
Master's	9	4.2%
Other degree	4	1.9%

Selecting "Include missing for grouping columns" causes Tabulate to display the counts and percentages of respondents that did not choose to supply the demographic information. In a survey, respondents commonly choose not to provide such demographic information for a variety of reasons such as fearing their opinions would become personally identifiable. In this survey only one of the nurses chose not to supply this information. From this summary, we see that staff nurses are the most frequently occurring organizational level, as would be expected. The distribution of years of service is fairly uniform, most of the nurses are employed on a full-time basis, and an associate's degree is the most frequently occurring educational level.

Figure 7.5 shows Distribution output for the survey responses to the question "There is sufficient information available for me to access when I have questions about the practice change." Note that the option has been selected to display a mosaic plot.

The histogram and mosaic plots show the nurses have widely varying opinions on this question, with nearly even splits between those that agree, disagree, and are neutral. Further analysis can be facilitated by creating a binary variable to combine those responses that agree with the proposition "There is sufficient information

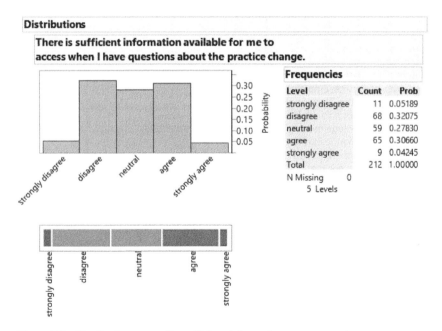

Figure 7.5 Distribution output for sufficient information survey question. (Analyze > Distribution. Highlight "There is sufficient information available for me to access when I have questions about the practice change" and click Y, Columns. Click OK. From the Distribution dropdown menu select Stack. Select Mosaic plot from option menu.)

Distributions

Sufficient Information

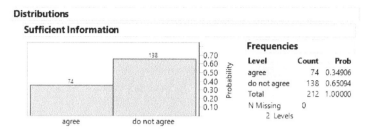

Frequencies

Level	Count	Prob
agree	74	0.34906
do not agree	138	0.65094
Total	212	1.00000
N Missing	0	

2 Levels

Figure 7.6 Distribution output for Sufficient Information column. (Analyze > Distribution. Highlight Sufficient Information and click Y, Columns. Click OK. From the Sufficient Information dropdown menu select Histogram Options > Show Counts.)

available for me to access when I have questions about the practice change" (agree and strongly agree responses) and those that do not agree (neutral, disagree, and strongly disagree). Neutral is categorized as "do not agree" since we have chosen to require an explicit affirmation of agreement. The JMP Recode feature can be used to create the column Sufficient Information using the method shown in Figure 7.3. The Distribution output for the binary variable Sufficient Information is shown in Figure 7.6. Note that the option has been selected to display the counts above the histogram bars.

When dichotomized, we find 65% of the nurses do not agree that there is sufficient information available, while 35% agree.

7.8.2 One-Sample Test of Proportion

It seems conclusive that there is insufficient nursing literature available for the nurses based on the 65% not in agreement. However, this conclusion is based on a sample of nurses' opinions and is subject to sampling error. A test of hypothesis for a proportion is an appropriate method to address the question "Do the majority of nurses feel that there is insufficient information available?" taking into account sampling error.

The first step in conducting a hypothesis test is to set up the null and alternative hypotheses. The null hypothesis assumes that the proportion of nurses who do not feel that the available information is sufficient is equal to 0.50. The alternative hypothesis can be specified in one of three ways, depending on the research question. A two-sided ($\neq$) alternative tests if the proportion in agreement differs from 0.50. There are two possible one-sided alternatives, less than or greater than 0.50. Since we are interested in determining if a majority of nurses do not agree that there is sufficient information, the appropriate alternative is a one-sided, greater than 0.50 alternative.

Once the null and alternative hypotheses are determined, the hypothesis test can be conducted with the JMP Distribution platform. Figure 7.7 shows the output.

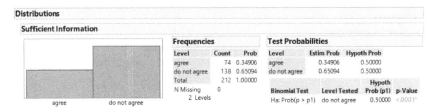

Figure 7.7 One-sample test of hypothesis for proportion results. (Analyze > Distribution. Select Test Probabilities from the Sufficient Information option menu. Enter 0.50 in the do not agree Hypoth Prob field; select the probabilities greater than hypothesized value radio button. Click Done.)

The key result is the *p*-value from the Binomial Test, which is <0.0001. The *p*-value is defined on a scale of 0 to 1 where small *p*-values cause a rejection of the null hypothesis and large *p*-values support the null hypothesis. The *p*-value is the likelihood of obtaining the sample proportion or something greater assuming the null hypothesis is true. In this case, the null hypothesis is rejected since the *p*-value of <0.0001 is less than 0.05, the chosen significance level. Therefore, we can conclude that a majority of nurses believe there is insufficient information available to them. Additional information on hypothesis testing can be found in Polit (2010) and Rosner (2015).

7.8.3 Test for Difference of Two Proportions

An objective of this analysis is to determine if the perception of the availability of sufficient information differs by organizational level (nurse leaders vs. staff nurses). Figure 7.8 shows the frequency of agreement for each of the two groups.

We see that there is only a small difference in the percentages between nurse leaders and staff nurses. However, establishing whether differences are statistically significant can only be done through a hypothesis test. For this situation, the null hypothesis is that the difference in proportions between the nurse leaders and staff nurses is equal to zero. A two-sided alternative is appropriate since we are looking for a difference between the two groups. To execute a test for two proportions in JMP, we use one of the options from the Fit Y by X platform. Figure 7.9 shows the relevant output.

Tabulate

| | Sufficient Information | | | |
| | agree | | do not agree | |
Org Level	N	Row %	N	Row %
Nurse Leader	9	36.00%	16	64.00%
Staff Nurse	64	34.41%	122	65.59%

Figure 7.8 Frequency for sufficient information by organization level. (Analyze > Tabulate. Drag Sufficient Information to the Drop zone for columns. Drag Org level to the Drop zone for rows. Drag Row % and N underneath Sufficient Information.)

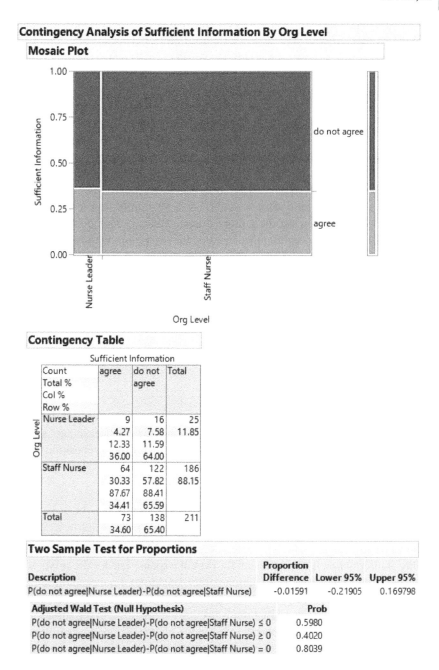

Contingency Analysis of Sufficient Information By Org Level

Mosaic Plot

Contingency Table

Sufficient Information

Count Total % Col % Row %	agree	do not agree	Total
Nurse Leader	9 4.27 12.33 36.00	16 7.58 11.59 64.00	25 11.85
Staff Nurse	64 30.33 87.67 34.41	122 57.82 88.41 65.59	186 88.15
Total	73 34.60	138 65.40	211

Two Sample Test for Proportions

Description	Proportion Difference	Lower 95%	Upper 95%
P(do not agree|Nurse Leader)-P(do not agree|Staff Nurse)	-0.01591	-0.21905	0.169798

Adjusted Wald Test (Null Hypothesis)	Prob
P(do not agree|Nurse Leader)-P(do not agree|Staff Nurse) $\leq$ 0	0.5980
P(do not agree|Nurse Leader)-P(do not agree|Staff Nurse) $\geq$ 0	0.4020
P(do not agree|Nurse Leader)-P(do not agree|Staff Nurse) = 0	0.8039

Figure 7.9 Two sample test of hypothesis for difference of proportions results. (Analyze > Fit Y by X. Enter Sufficient Information as the Y, Response and Org Level as the X, Factor. Click OK. From the Contingency Analysis option menu, select Two Sample Test for Proportions.)

The mosaic plot by Org Level shows visually that the two groups have a similar opinion on this question. The width of the column in the mosaic plot is proportional to the sample size for each group. The smaller mosaic plot to the right shows percentages for all respondents taken together. The Contingency Table shows the relative frequencies overall and conditional on row (Org Level) and column (Sufficient Information). The Two Sample Test for Proportions output shows the difference in the sample proportions (−0.016) and a 95% confidence interval on that difference. The 95% confidence interval gives a range of plausible values for the true difference in proportions. We are 95% confident that the true difference in proportions lies between −0.22 and 0.17. The *p*-values associated with the three possible alternative hypotheses follow. Since we have chosen a two-sided alternative, the corresponding *p*-value is 0.8039. At a 5% significance level, there is insufficient evidence to reject the null hypothesis. We can conclude that there is no statistically significance difference between the two groups with respect to the proportion who feel the availability of information is insufficient for their needs. When the confidence interval contains 0, this means that there is no significant difference. Additional explanation on tests for the difference of proportions can be found in Polit (2010) and Rosner (2015).

7.9 Summary

7.9.1 Statistical Insights

Analysis of the survey results for the question "There is sufficient information available for me to access when I have questions about the practice change" shows that approximately 65% of the nurses do not agree with this proposition. This response is consistent for both staff nurses and nurse managers. Statistical tests of hypothesis established these conclusions.

7.9.2 Implications and Next Steps

While a clear majority of both staff nurses and nurse leaders feel that the availability of information is not sufficient, the overall response rate for the survey was only 25%. Since the survey was voluntary, this constitutes a nonrandom sample and as such leaves open the possibility of self-selection bias influencing the results. It may be reasonably assumed that those electing to participate in the survey may hold stronger opinions, either positive or negative, about the nursing environment and pursuit of magnet certification than those who chose not to participate. Other reasons for nonresponse may include fear of retaliation from supervisors based on the possibility of responses being personally identifiable or technology issues with accessing or completing the survey. Conclusions drawn from this analysis must be tempered by the participation rates and potential biases. Applying principles of good survey design and administration can help mitigate issues associated with bias and response rates (Babbie, 2015).

As a next step, the Nursing Research and Evidence-based Practice Council could consider the use of focus groups, randomly selected from both nurse leaders and staff nurses, to help validate the survey results and to obtain more detailed information on specific actions that can be taken to improve the availability of nursing research information. For example, the hospital may not be subscribing to journals in a specific field of nursing or the assistance of a librarian may not be available to nurses working on the evening shift. Additionally, as a part of the benchmarking process, it may be possible to ascertain if nurses at other hospitals share the same level of agreement regarding sufficiency of nursing research information.

7.9.3 Summary of Tools and JMP Features

Statistical methods tools	Data management concepts	JMP platform features	Quality tools
Descriptive statistics	Missing data	Cols > Columns Viewer	Benchmarking
– Histogram – Mosaic plot		Tables > Missing Data Pattern	Voice of the customer
Hypothesis test for one proportion	Derived data		Surveys
Hypothesis test for the difference of two proportions		Cols > Recode	
Confidence interval		Tabulate Distribution Fit Y by X	

7.9.4 Exercises

1. Repeat the two sample test of proportion analysis shown in this case comparing the perceptions of full time and part time/per diem nurses. Write a paragraph that summarizes the results.

2. Explore the alternative for summarizing categorical variables by repeating the descriptive analysis for the rating question on sufficiency of information using Analyze > Consumer Research > Categorical. Compare the summary to that given in the case.

3. Repeat the analysis from this case for the question "Literature and research findings are useful in my daily practice." (You will need to create a new column that dichotomizes the responses.) How do the results compare with those for the question analyzed in this case?

4. A confidence interval is a statistical inference procedure that allows you to determine a range of plausible values for a parameter such as the mean or the proportion.

   (a) Compute a 95% confidence interval for the proportion of nurses that agreed that there was sufficient information available. Give a brief interpretation of this confidence interval.

   (b) Compare the confidence interval to the test of hypothesis. Explain the difference between them and suggest when it is appropriate to use each method.

5. Are the responses to the two questions "Literature and research finds are useful in my daily practice" and "There is sufficient information available for me to access when I have questions about the practice change" associated?

   (a) Conduct a χ^2 test for independence and interpret the results.

   (b) Display a table of association measures by selecting "Measures of Association" from the Contingency Analysis options menu. Report the Gamma and Kendall's Tau-b measures and briefly explain how these measures are calculated and how they differ.

7.9.5 Discussion Questions

1. In the nurses' survey, nearly 25% of the respondents either did not respond to any survey questions or chose not to provide demographic information. Discuss possible reasons for these nonresponses. Research best practices in survey design and administration that could help to mitigate nonresponse.

2. Survey participants often worry that their responses can be personally identified by their demographic characteristics. What methods are used in data analysis and survey administration to prevent survey responses from being personally identified.

3. Find and share examples of survey results that are presented to the general public. Critically evaluate the presentations, identifying strengths and weaknesses.

References

Babbie, E. (2015). *The Practice of Social Research*, 14e. Cengage Learning.

Gale, B.V.P. and Schaffer, M.A. (2009). Organizational readiness for evidenced-based practice. *Journal of Nursing Administration* 39 (2): 91–97.

Polit, D.F. (2010). *Statistics and Data Analysis for Nursing Research*, 2e. Pearson.

Rosner, B. (2015). *Fundamentals of Biostatistics*, 8e. Cengage Learning.

8

Determining the Sample Size for a Nursing Research Study

8.1 Key Concepts

Sample size determination, study design, power analysis, hypothesis testing.

8.2 DMAIC

I: In this case, you will use tools that apply to the Improve phase in the Define–Measure–Analyze–Improve–Control (DMAIC) process.

8.3 PDCA

P: In this case, you will use tools that apply to the Plan step in the Plan–Do–Check–Act (PDCA) process.

8.4 Background

Nurses at a suburban urgent care facility in Upstate New York discovered a published study (Müller et al 2011) showing that topical application of heat for treating bee/wasp stings relieved symptoms more quickly than cold, the current standard of care. A literature search showed very few studies that compared the effectiveness of heat vs. cold therapy. Seeking to improve the quality of patient care, the nurses proposed a clinical intervention study. The purpose of this study was to learn to what extent the application of topical heat or cold impacted patients'

Improving Health Care Quality: Case Studies with JMP®, First Edition.
Mary Ann Shifflet, Cecilia Martinez, Jane Oppenlander, and Shirley Shmerling.
© 2020 John Wiley & Sons, Inc. Published 2020 by John Wiley & Sons, Inc.
Books Companion site:www.wiley.com/go/shifflet/improvinghealthcarequality1e

experiences of pain, swelling, and itchiness after a bee or wasp sting. With the endorsement of their management, two nurses, supported by an experienced nursing researcher and a statistician, spearheaded the design of the study.

Quality improvement initiatives often utilize designed studies to evaluate the efficacy of process or clinical changes. This case illustrates one important aspect of study design, how to determine appropriate sample size.

8.5   The Task

Determine an appropriate sample size for a clinical intervention study that compares the effectiveness of heat vs. cold therapy for relieving symptoms of bee/wasp stings.

8.6   The Data

In order to determine an appropriate sample size for the study, the nurses identified pain, swelling, and itchiness as measurable factors that led to patient discomfort at the site of a bee/wasp sting. They planned to measure these symptoms using previously validated, reliable scales. Pain would be measured using the Wong Pain Faces scale and itchiness with the visual analog scale (VAS). Both of these are ordinal scales. Swelling would be measured in centimeters at its longest extent at the sting site.

The number of patients treated for bee stings at the urgent care in the previous two calendar years was also obtained.

8.7   Study Design and Data Collection Methodology

The study team prepared the intervention protocol, designed a data collection tool for the nurses to use when evaluating patients, developed a data management and analysis plan, and conducted training sessions for the nurses. An important aspect of their preparation was to complete the research project proposal and informed consent forms to obtain approval from their institutional review board (IRB). United States federal law requires that organizations conducting biomedical or behavioral research have an IRB that evaluates research studies to ensure the protection of human subjects.

The study was designed so that a patient meeting the eligibility requirements and consenting to participate was randomly assigned to receive either the hot or cold therapy. Large envelopes containing either a cold or hot pack, a data collection sheet, and other equipment needed to treat a patient, were randomized in blocks of four (two cold packs and two hot packs per block) and placed in a container. Block randomization ensures that balance will be maintained between the number of cold and hot therapy subjects over time. A balanced experiment is one that has the same number of test subjects in each treatment group. A nurse needing a treatment packet would take the next envelope in sequence from the container. The envelopes were opaque and not marked as to whether a cold or hot pack was contained inside.

The team planned a small pilot study to test the data collection method and treatment protocol. The research proposal required the specification of the study duration and the number of patients that would need to participate to obtain statistically valid results.

8.8 Analysis

8.8.1 Analysis Plan

Before the study began, an analysis plan was developed to assure that the necessary data was collected and could be efficiently transcribed from the paper data collection sheet to an electronic form. The pilot study not only included the clinical protocol but also the data transcription and statistical analysis. A comprehensive pilot study covering all aspects of a study is a best practice. This helps assure efficient protocol execution and data collection and analysis to address the research questions. Frequently, pilot studies uncover issues, that if left uncorrected, can lead to rework or reduced data quantity or quality.

The differences between the changes in pain and itchiness before and after treatment for the hot and cold therapy pilot groups were evaluated using a Mann–Whitney U test (in JMP® referred to as a Wilcoxon test) since they are ordinal measures. For further detail on this test see Rosner (2015). The extent of swelling change between the two treatments was evaluated using a two-independent samples t-test. This test was used as the basis for the sample size determination.

Finally, the analysis plan called for a retrospective analysis of the prior two calendar years to see how many patients were treated for bee stings each year. A total of 61 and 100 patients meeting the study's inclusion criteria were treated for bee stings in the prior two years, respectively. Information from past years will help guide the sample size selection. In addition, the analysis showed that no bee stings were treated during the winter months of December through February. This knowledge assisted the team in their project planning so that they were prepared to begin the study in March.

8.8.2 The Basics of Sample Size Determination

In this study, we want to determine if there is a significant difference in the extent of swelling at the sting site as a result of the two therapies. In addition, changes in pain and itchiness will be evaluated. For the remainder of this case, we will focus on the extent of swelling. A two-independent samples t-test is an appropriate method to determine if a statistically significant difference exists between the average change in swelling for the two groups.

In statistical hypothesis testing, null and alternative hypotheses are posed to correspond to a research question. Data is collected and sample estimates are used to either support or refute the null hypothesis. Sample size determination is directly related to the specification of the hypothesis test. There are four values that are needed to determine sample size: detectable difference, an estimate of the process standard deviation, significance level, and power. Each of these values is explained later.

Sample estimates are subject to variation. Two types of errors can occur in hypothesis testing that can lead to incorrect conclusions. A Type I error (with probability α) occurs when the null hypothesis is rejected when it is in fact true. This is analogous to a "false positive" on a screening test for a disease where a person tests positive, but actually does not have the disease. This probability is often referred to as the significance level. Typically, Type I errors are set to 0.05, although values from 0.01 to 0.10 are common. Study investigators choose the values for these errors before the study begins, based on their risk tolerance for making an incorrect conclusion.

A Type II error (with probability β) occurs if the null hypothesis is not rejected, when the alternative is in fact true. This is analogous to a "false negative" on a screening test for a disease where a person tests negative, but actually has the disease. The power of a test is defined as $(1 - \beta)$ or the probability that there is evidence to support the alternative hypothesis when it is in fact true. In biomedical studies, tests with relatively high powers are desired, as this assures that differences between treatment outcomes will be detected, if they exist, with high probability. Typical values for power are 0.80 to 0.95. Power analysis is conducted prior to beginning a study to find the sample size needed to assure that an effect can be detected, if it exists, with relatively high power. The situations leading to each of the hypothesis testing errors are illustrated in Figure 8.1.

The difference to detect must be chosen by investigators to specify the size of the effect they wish to discover. For example, the investigators could be interested in detecting a difference of 0.5 cm in the average extent of swelling between the two groups. The choice of the difference to detect is related to a meaningful or practical difference between the two groups. For example, a difference of 0.1 cm

Possible hypothesis test outcomes		
	Actual situation	
Decision	H_0 true Parameter = Benchmark	H_0 false Parameter ≠ Benchmark (or other option)
Do not reject H_0	No error probability $1 - \alpha$	Type II error Probability β
Reject H_0	Type I error Probability α	No error Probability $1 - \beta$

Figure 8.1 Hypothesis testing errors.

in the average swelling may not be a sufficiently large clinical difference to warrant changing the standard therapy from cold to hot.

Finally, an estimate of the process standard deviation is needed for sample size determination. An estimate can be obtained from the literature, clinical expertise, or a pilot study. Additional details on hypothesis test and sample size determination can be found in Rosner (2015) and Polit (2010).

8.8.3 Sample Size Determination for the Bee Sting Study

The nurses chose a difference to detect for change in swelling of 1 cm. From their clinical experience, they estimated the standard deviation of the change in swelling associated with the cold therapy to be 1.5 cm. They felt that it would be reasonable to assume that the standard deviation would be the same for the hot therapy based on both their clinical experience and literature review. Initially, they chose a significance level (α) of 0.05 and power ($1 - \beta$) of 0.90.

The JMP Sample Size and Power dialog, shown in Figure 8.2, allows the user to select the sample size calculation corresponding to the desired statistical test that will be performed.

For this example, select Two Sample Means and complete the dialog as shown in Figure 8.3a. Clicking Continue will produce the sample size result shown in Figure 8.3b.

Given the historical frequency of bee stings for the prior two years (61 and 100 cases), the project team decided that a sample size of 97 is too large, and they desired a smaller sample size. Subsequently, sample sizes were calculated for several combinations of power and difference to detect. This is done by clearing the Sample Size field and modifying values in the Difference to Detect and Power fields. Ultimately, the project settled on a sample size of 73 where the significance level was 0.05, the power was 0.80, and the difference to detect was 1 cm.

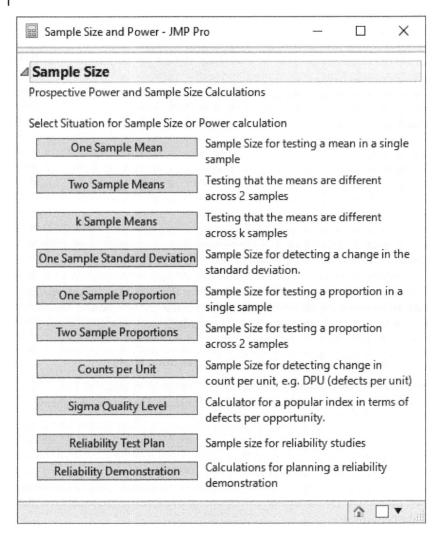

Figure 8.2 JMP Sample Size and Power dialog.
(DOE > Design Diagnostics > Sample Size and Power.)

Continuing the power analysis, the project team wanted to ascertain what differences could be detected based on the historical frequency of bee stings. This can be found by specifying the Sample Size, Power, and Alpha and leaving the Difference to detect field blank. Table 8.1 shows the results for sample sizes of 60 and 100.

While the project team chose a sample size of 73, they realized that the number of patients who seek treatment could be less than that based on the historical frequencies. Table 8.1 shows that if only 60 samples were obtained, the difference

Sample Size

┌─Two Means─────────────────────────────┐
Testing if two means are different from each other.
Alpha   0.05
Std Dev   1.5
Extra Parameters   0

Supply two values to determine the third.
Enter one value to see a plot of the other two.

Difference to detect   1
Sample Size   .
Power   .
Sample Size is the total sample size; per group would be n/2
Continue
Back

Sample Size

┌─Two Means─────────────────────────────┐
Testing if two means are different from each other.
Alpha   0.05
Std Dev   1.5
Extra Parameters   0

Supply two values to determine the third.
Enter one value to see a plot of the other two.

Difference to detect   1
Sample Size   97
Power   0.9
Sample Size is the total sample size; per group would be n/2
Continue
Back

(a)   (b)

Figure 8.3 JMP Sample Size and Power calculations for two sample means.

Table 8.1 Differences to detect for various sample sizes.

Sample size	Alpha	Power	Standard deviation	Difference to detect (cm)
60	0.05	0.80	1.5	1.1
100	0.05	0.80	1.5	0.85

that could be detected was 1.1 cm. The project team was comfortable that the results would be meaningful if a sample size of only 60 was obtained.

An alternative approach is to use the JMP Sample Size and Power feature to produce a graph, called a power curve, which shows the relationship between sample size and difference to detect. Figure 8.4 shows a power curve for this case.

In general, fixing any three parameters and leaving the other two parameter fields blank in the Sample Size and Power dialog will yield a curve showing the relationship between those two parameters. Figure 8.5 shows the relationship between Sample Size and Power.

8.9 Summary

8.9.1 Statistical Insights

Appropriate sample sizes for a study are determined by the significance level, power, difference to detect, and an estimate of the process standard deviation. A sample size calculated for a desired significance level, power, and difference to detect may be larger than is practical to achieve. For example, resources are

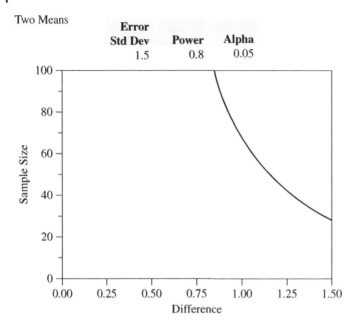

Figure 8.4 Power curve for Sample Size and Difference to detect for bee sting study. (DOE > Design Diagnostics > Sample Size and Power. Enter 0.05 for Alpha, 1.5 for Std Dev, 0 for Extra Parameters, and 0.80 for Power. (Leave Difference to Detect and Sample Size blank). Click Continue.)

unavailable or in this case, there was a likelihood that the desired sample size may not be reached based on the number of patients treated for bee stings in the two previous years. The use of the JMP sample size calculator (as shown in Figures 8.2 and 8.3) allowed the research team to find sample sizes associated with various combinations of significance level, power, and difference to detect. In addition, a sensitivity analysis (Table 8.1) showed the differences that could be detected for various sample sizes and provided assurance that the results would be acceptable for sample sizes somewhat lower than desired. This gave the research team confidence that the study would produce valid results given the uncertainty in the number of future patients that will be treated for bee stings.

8.9.2 Implications and Next Steps

Sample size determination is an important aspect of experiment/study design that should be conducted prior to beginning a study to be sure that the objectives can be reached with the available resources. Having an estimate of the number of study subjects is needed when preparing project plans and budgets. In addition, when human subjects are involved, IRBs may require a sample size calculation or power

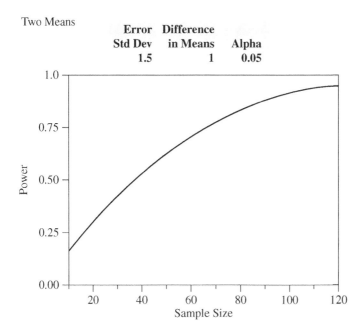

Figure 8.5 Power curve for Sample Size and Power for bee sting study. (DOE > Design Diagnostics > Sample Size and Power. Enter 0.05 for Alpha, 1.5 for Std Dev, 0 for Extra Parameters, and 1 for Difference to Detect. (Leave Sample Size and Power blank). Click Continue.)

analysis be included in the materials submitted to be sure that statistically valid conclusions can be drawn (Table 8.2).

8.9.3 Summary of Tools and JMP Features

Table 8.2 Summary of Tools and JMP Features.

Statistical methods tools	Data management concepts	JMP platform features	Quality tools
Hypothesis test		DOE > Sample and size and power	Assessing variation
Sample size determination			Experimental/study design
Power analysis			

8.9.4 Exercises

1. Repeat the sample size calculations for this case using α of 0.01. Compare the results with those when α was 0.05.
2. Find sample sizes for $\alpha = 0.05$, difference to detect = 1, and powers of 0.8 to 0.95 in increments of 0.05. Describe how sample size changes as power changes.
3. Find samples sizes for $\alpha = 0.05$, power = 0.9, and differences to detect of 0.5 to 2 cm in increments of 0.5 cm. Describe how sample size changes as difference to detect changes.
4. What differences could be detected for sample sizes of 24, 35, 50, and 100? Use $\alpha = 0.05$ and power = 0.90.
5. Create a power curve for difference to detect and power for a sample size of 73. Explain what this power curve tells an investigator.
6. Some healthcare organizations do not have statistical software available. In such cases, sample size calculators are available on the Internet. Search the Internet for a sample size calculator and use it to calculate the sample size for the bee sting study as shown in this case. Compare the features and usability of this online calculator to JMP's capabilities.

8.9.5 Discussion Questions

1. Find a published medical study on a topic of your choice. Prepare a brief summary of the study objectives, data collection method, the study population, inclusion and exclusion criteria, and the sample size. Comment on these aspects of the study, identifying strengths and weaknesses in the published article.
2. Research the topic of effect size. Explain how it is related to hypothesis testing and sample size determination. Give an example of a study where effect size is discussed.
3. US federal law requires protection of human subjects involved in biomedical and behavioral research. IRBs are required to review and approve proposed studies to ensure human subjects are properly protected. Obtain a copy of the forms that must be submitted to your organization's IRB. Alternatively, you can search the Internet for a sample proposal form. Evaluate the forms and discuss how sample size is reported. Why is it important for an IRB to review sample size associated with a medical study?
4. Informed consent is another provision to protect human subjects involved in biomedical and behavioral research. Research the concept of informed consent and prepare a brief summary of what informed consent is and why it is needed.

Discuss how obtaining consent relates to determining sample size when designing a study.

5. Discuss the concept of practical vs. statistical significance. Search the literature and find examples to share. How can practical significance be determined?

References

Müller, B., Großjohann, C., and Fischer, L. (2011). The use of concentrated heat after insect bites/stings as an alternative to reduce swelling, pain, and pruritus: an open cohort-study at German beaches and bathing-lakes. *Clinical, Cosmetic and Investigational Dermatology* 4: 191–196.

Polit, D.F. (2010). *Statistics and Data Analysis for Nursing Research*, 2e. Pearson.

Rosner, B. (2015). *Fundamentals of Biostatistics*, 8e. Cengage Learning.

9
Mapping California Ambulance Diversion

9.1   Key Concepts

Descriptive statistics, Data visualization, mapping, data cleaning.

9.2   DMAIC

A: The tools illustrated in this case are frequently applied in the Analyze phase of the Define–Measure–Analyze–Improve–Control (DMAIC) approach to process improvement.

9.3   PDCA

PA: In this case, you will use tools that apply to the Plan and Act steps in the Plan–Do–Check–Act (PDCA) process.

9.4   Background

Hospital emergency departments (EDs) employ ambulance diversion as a temporary measure to relieve patient flow issues by sending ambulances transporting patients that are not seriously ill to another facility. This may be necessary when overcrowding occurs in the ED or when there are no inpatient beds available for ED patients that require hospital admission. Ambulance diversion can reduce the quality of patient care, increase wait times for treatment, reduce availability of

Improving Health Care Quality: Case Studies with JMP®, First Edition.
Mary Ann Shifflet, Cecilia Martinez, Jane Oppenlander, and Shirley Shmerling.
© 2020 John Wiley & Sons, Inc. Published 2020 by John Wiley & Sons, Inc.
Books Companion site:www.wiley.com/go/shifflet/improvinghealthcarequality1e

ambulances, and cause loss of hospital revenue. The key performance metric is the number of hours an ED is on ambulance diversion, meaning they are not accepting any new ED patients by ambulance.

Ambulance diversion, once a temporary measure, has become routine for many hospitals, particularly those in urban areas and those that are trauma centers. Factors contributing to the increase in ambulance diversion are increasing demand for emergency medical services (EMS), lack of coordination between local EMS dispatching agencies, and decreased emergency department capacities. A number of initiatives have been undertaken to address this issue, notably the California Emergency Department Diversion Project (California Healthcare Foundation, 2009).

In this case, we will examine the extent of ambulance diversion at California general acute care hospitals for 2015. An initial understanding of the variation and potential causes for ambulance diversion is valuable in the early stages of a quality improvement initiative. Efficient management of emergency department patient flow can improve the quality of patient care, increase efficiency in operations at the hospital and regional levels, and reduce healthcare costs.

9.5   The Task

The objective of this case is to visualize the variation in total 2015 ambulance diversion hours for general acute care hospitals in California by creating maps.

9.6   The Data: ED_ambulance_diversion_trend.xlsx and CA_healthcare_facility_locations.xlsx

The California Health and Human Services Agency makes nonconfidential data available to the public from their open data portal. The file ED_ambulance _diversion_trend.xlsx was downloaded from this portal and contains hospital level information on ambulance diversion for the years 2007 through 2015. The file CA_healthcare_facility_locations.xlsx contains information on the locations and characteristics of California healthcare facilities and was also downloaded from the portal. Data definitions for both of these files can be found in the downloadable data dictionaries (California Health and Human Services Agency, n.d.) and are provided with the data files that accompany this casebook.

9.7   Data Management

Several data processing steps are needed to prepare the files for analysis.

9.7.1 Merging the Data Tables

To begin, the two data files need to be merged to associate the geographic location data for each hospital (latitude and longitude) with the corresponding ambulance diversion hours. The California Health and Human Services Agency has designed their files so that some contain general hospital characteristics, such as bed capacity and location, and others have more specific information such as frequency of hospital-acquired conditions, financial performance, and ambulance diversion hours. This is a best practice in data management as files can be merged as needed to address specific analyses and data is maintained in only one location.

Open both data files in JMP® (CA_healthcare_facility_locations.xlsx and ED_ambulance_diversion_trend.xlsx). Two or more data sheets can be "joined" through a common column in each table. Figure 9.1 shows the completed join dialog where the name of the facility is the common column.

Save the file as CA_ambulance_diversion_2015_raw.jmp. A column called "Match Flag" has been added that shows the match result of the join performed. For this join, the value "Both" is found in all rows of this column indicating that the data was found in both tables.

Prior to selecting the join columns, it is important to be sure that they contain exactly the same information. There are different types of Join operations (inner join and several types of outer joins) and options that can be selected to handle nonmatching rows. Additional information on joining JMP data tables can be found in the Reshape Data section of the book Using JMP which can be accessed from Help > Books > Using JMP (2018).

9.7.2 Reviewing the Merged File

JMP's Columns Viewer is an easy way to do an initial review of the merged data file to discover issues such as columns of duplicated information (as would be the case when column names do not match), missing data, columns that should be assigned a different JMP modeling type, and other data anomalies. Figure 9.2 shows a portion of the Columns Viewer output for the merged file. Familiarity with the data dictionaries will facilitate the interpretation of the Columns Viewer results.

After reviewing the Columns Viewer output, a number of modifications to the merged data table are needed, including changing JMP modeling types. For example, Year should be changed from continuous to ordinal since the mean and standard deviation are not meaningful. In addition, there are columns of duplicate information that can be deleted.

Both files contained information on the trauma center level designation with one file having a value of 0 for hospitals that are not trauma centers, while the other

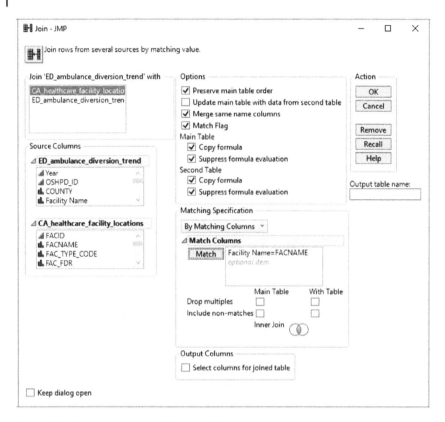

Figure 9.1 Dialog to join two JMP data tables.
(Tables > Join. Select CA_healthcare_facility_locations in the Join with field. Select Facility Name and FACNAME from the Source Columns field. Check Merge same column names. Click Match. Click OK.)

file left the cells blank. There are however, discrepancies between the information in the two files. For example, the Trauma Ctr Designation column indicates that 120 of the hospitals are Level I, while the column TRAUMA_CTR identifies 61 Level I hospitals. This discrepancy must be resolved before proceeding with the analysis. In practice, this would require consultation with the data owner. For this case, we will use the Trauma Ctr Designation column.

Another example of data that needs to be "cleaned up" is the column Ambulance Diversion Reported, which is an indicator variable and as shown in Figure 9.3 has three categories. Figure 9.3 shows JMP Distribution output for this variable which reveals a data anomaly that can be corrected with the JMP Recode feature (Highlight the column Ambulance Diversion Reported, then select Cols > Recode). In addition, unneeded columns, such as hospital contact information can be deleted.

⊿ ▾ Summary Statistics

68 Columns Clear Select Distribution

Columns	N	N Missing	N Categories	Min	Max	Mean	Std Dev
Match Flag	2491	0	1				
Year	2491	0	.	2007	2015	2011.2994781	2.588093631072
OSHPD_ID	2491	0	.	106010735	206351814	106847209.43	7475236.825477
COUNTY	2491	0	96				
Facility Name	2491	0	316				
Address	2491	0	348				
City	2491	0	206				
ZIP Code	2491	0	303				
Trauma Ctr Designation	2491	0	5				
Trauma Ctr Designation Pediatric	2491	0	3				
EMS Level January 1st	2491	0	4				
EMS Level December 31st	2491	0	4				
EMS Visits Total	2491	0	.	0	168351	26698.571658	28014.79984038
EMS Visits Total - Admitted	2491	0	.	0	35835	4151.0393416	4881.541478929
EMS Treatment Stations	2488	3	.	0	116	15.599678457	17.04299631104
EMS Non-emergent Visits	2491	0	.	0	77883	2146.7073464	7850.126250172
EMS Registered Without Treatment	2491	0	.	0	31407	787.39020474	1673.890923442
Ambulance Diversion Reported	2491	0	3				
January	2491	0	.	0	532	31.246085909	76.28492918933
February	2491	0	.	0	534	27.298273786	69.93207657698

Figure 9.2 Columns Viewer output for merged ambulance diversion file.
(Cols> Columns Viewer. Select all columns in the Select Columns field. Click Show Summary.)

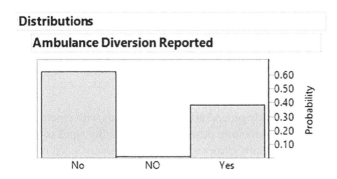

Distributions

Ambulance Diversion Reported

Frequencies

Level	Count	Prob
No	1544	0.61983
NO	10	0.00401
Yes	937	0.37615
Total	2491	1.00000
N Missing	0	

3 Levels

Figure 9.3 Distribution output for Ambulance Diversion Reported.
(Highlight Ambulance Diversion Reported in the Summary Statistics table. Click Distribution.)

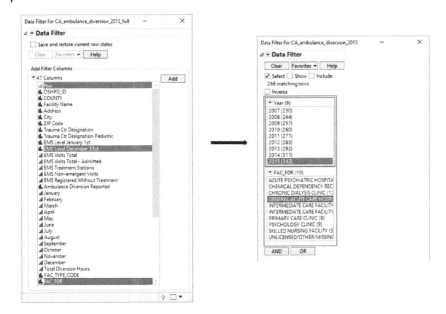

Figure 9.4 Data Filter dialog to select general acute care hospitals. (Rows > Data Filter. Highlight Year, EMS Level December 31st, and FAC_FDR, in the Add Filter Columns field and click Add. Select the highlighted values in the resulting field. Tables > Subset.)

9.7.3 Extracting General Acute Care Hospital Data

The scope of this case includes only general acute care hospitals with emergency departments for the year 2015. Data from other healthcare facility types such as skilled nursing facilities and specialty clinics and other years are included in this file. In addition, hospitals that have a value of 0 for EMS Level do not have emergency departments; these hospitals should not be included. The JMP Data Filter can be used to create a JMP data table containing only the 2015 information for general acute care hospitals with emergency departments as shown in Figure 9.4.

The cleaned file has been saved as CA_ambulance_diversion_2015.jmp with a total of 221 hospitals.

9.8 Analysis

9.8.1 Descriptive Analysis

Always begin an analysis by familiarizing yourself with the key variables using descriptive statistics and data visualizations. Figure 9.5 shows the Distribution output for Total Diversion Hours and Ambulance Diversion Reported.

Distributions

Total Diversion Hours

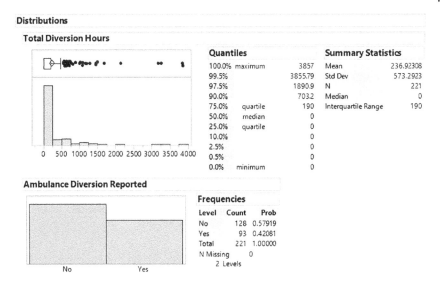

Ambulance Diversion Reported

Figure 9.5 Summary statistics for Total Diversion Hours and Ambulance Diversion Reported.
(Analyze > Distribution. Drag the two variables of interest to the Y, Columns field. Click OK. From the Distribution dropdown menu select Stack. From the Summary Statistics dropdown menu select Customize Summary Statistics and select the statistics shown.)

The analysis shows that 57.9% of hospitals did not report any ambulance diversion during 2015. To analyze the Total Diversion Hours for only those hospitals reporting ambulance diversion click on the "No" bar in the Ambulance Diversion Reported bar chart. In the data table, select Rows > Exclude/Unexclude to exclude the hospitals with no diversion from the summary. The Distribution output for Total Diversion Hours excluding those hospitals that had no ambulance diversion is shown in Figure 9.6.

Total diversion hours ranged from 1 to 3857 for those hospitals reporting ambulance diversion with a median of 302 hours and an interquartile range of 611 hours. Median and interquartile range are the preferred measures of centrality and variation, respectively, for skewed distributions.

9.8.2   Geographic Distribution of Total Diversion Hours

Additional insight into ambulance diversion in California can be gained by mapping Total Diversion Hours using JMP's Graph Builder. Each hospital's location is given by its latitude and longitude. Figure 9.7 shows the hospitals plotted on a map with the size of the marker corresponding to the number of diversion hours.

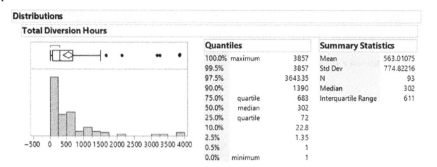

Figure 9.6 Summary statistics for Total Diversion Hours for hospitals reporting ambulance diversion.
(To refresh the analysis for Total Diversion Hours from the output window click on the Distribution dropdown menu, select Redo > Automatic Recalc.)

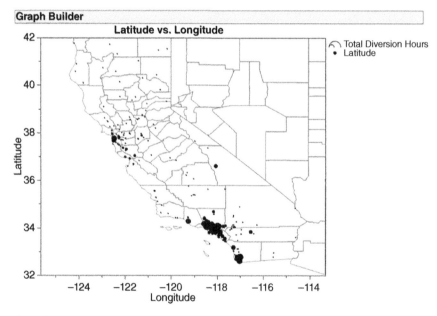

Figure 9.7 Map of Total Diversion Hours.
(Drag Latitude to the Y drop zone. Drag Longitude to the X drop zone. Drag Total Diversion Hours to the Size drop zone. Right click over one of the markers and select Graph > Background map. Select US Counties from the Boundaries list. Click OK. Click Done.)

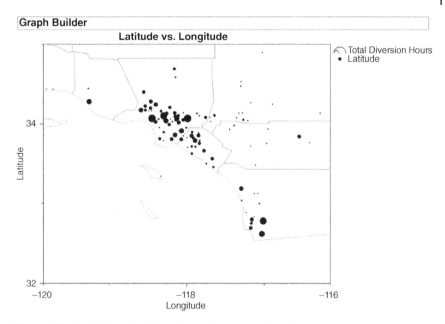

Figure 9.8 Total Diversion Hours for southern coastal region.
(Left Click *x*-axis. Select Axis Settings. Change Minimum to -120 and Maximum to -116.
Click OK. Left click *y*-axis. Select Axis Settings. Change Minimum to 32 and Maximum to 35. Click OK.)

This map shows a larger concentration of hospitals on the coast near the major cities of San Francisco, Los Angeles, and San Diego and that the most ambulance diversion occurs in these areas, particularly in the Los Angeles region. In the less densely populated areas of the state, hospitals are farther apart, making ambulance diversion impractical.

To zoom into the southern coastal region (Los Angeles and San Diego), change the bounds of the *x*- and *y*-axis scales as shown in Figure 9.8.

Some hospitals are designated as trauma centers, meaning they have advanced capabilities for caring for trauma patients. Nationally, there are four levels of trauma care with Level IV centers having the highest capability for treating trauma patients. Figure 9.9 shows the southern coastal region map with the trauma center level added on a color scale. This map shows that in this region there is a wide variation in ambulance diversion hours regardless of trauma center designation.

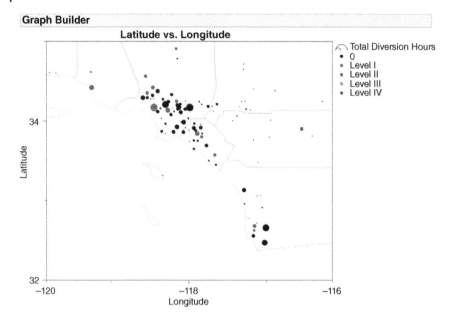

Figure 9.9 Map of Total Diversion Hours and Trauma Ctr Designation.
(Continuing from Figure 9.8 drag Trauma Ctr Designation to the Color drop zone.)

9.9 Summary

9.9.1 Statistical Insights

The maps created in this case clearly show that ambulance diversion occurs in metropolitan areas where there are high population densities and multiple hospitals in close proximity. There does not appear to be any relationship between a hospital's trauma center designation and ambulance diversion. These maps suggest that ambulance diversion is being used to alleviate ED overcrowding when there are other hospitals in close proximity. These insights would not be evident from other commonly used visualizations such as histograms. Further statistical tests can be applied to definitively determine if a relationship exists.

9.9.2 Implications and Next Steps

Geographic visualizations are useful, when applicable, in the Analyze phase of the DMAIC process when assessing variability, identifying potential causes of ambulance diversion, and prioritizing the need to reduce ambulance diversion at a particular hospital. Maps allow multivariate visualization through the use of color and size scales. Such visualizations are key tools that can assist healthcare quality improvement initiatives in developing strategies to alleviate ED overcrowding as one part of the overall objective of improving hospital patient flow. They also serve as means to communicate geospatial data to a wide audience.

9.9.3 Summary of Tools and JMP Features

Statistical methods tools	Data management concepts	JMP platform features	Quality tools
Descriptive statistics	Joining	Tables > Join	Assessing variation
Data visualization	Subsetting	Data filter	
– Histogram			
– Map			
		Recode	
		Distribution	
		Graph Builder	

9.9.4 Exercises

1. Prepare a statistical summary (i.e., tables of descriptive statistics and graphs) from the case data that describes the characteristics of the California hospitals (e.g., bed capacity, ownership, etc.)
2. Recreate the map shown in Figure 9.7 but instead of using US county boundaries as the background map, choose the image "Simple Earth."
   (a) Change the background map to the image "Detailed Earth."
   (b) What additional information is provided by using an image as a background map?
   (c) Which of the three background maps do you feel is most effective in this situation? Explain the rationale for your choice.
3. Create a map of total diversion hours that focuses on San Francisco and the Bay Area. Add another variable of your choice as a color scale. Write a few sentences to compare this map with the map of the Los Angeles area found in this case.
4. Create a map of California hospitals that shows diversion hours and add bed capacity with a color scale. How does this map add insight into the problem of ambulance diversion?
5. Create an alternate visualization (not a map) that shows total diversion hours by trauma center designation.
   (a) What does this visualization tell you about the relationship between trauma center designation and total diversion hours?

(b) Use Tabulate to create a table of descriptive statistics for total diversion hours by trauma center designation.

(c) What is the appropriate statistical method to determine if there are significant differences in mean total diversion hours for trauma center designations I, II, III, and IV? Conduct the analysis and summarize your findings in one page or less.

6. The file CA_ambulance_diversion_2007_2015.jmp contains ambulance diversion data for California general acute care hospitals for the years 2007–2015. Create a series of maps by year. This can be done by dragging Year into the Page drop zone in Graph Builder. Comment on how ambulance diversion changes over this nine-year period.

9.9.5 Discussion Questions

1. Select two hospitals in close geographic proximity, one that experiences ambulance diversions and one that does not. Conduct research to understand the characteristics of these hospitals and their surrounding communities. Identify potential reasons why one hospital experiences ambulance diversions and the other does not.

2. Conduct an Internet/literature search to identify the consequences of ambulance diversion on the quality of patient care and associated health outcomes. What are the consequences of ambulance diversion on hospital operations? Are hospitals conducting quality improvement initiatives to address these issues?

3. Search the Internet for examples where maps are used to display information. Discuss the intended audience for these visualizations and why they are effective communication tools.

References

California Healthcare Foundation (2009, July). California ED Diversion Project. Final Report. Retrieved from: http://www.caeddiversionproject.com/.

California Health and Human Services Agency (n.d.) California Health and Human Services Data Portal. Retrieved from https://data.chhs.ca.gov/

JMP (2018). *Using JMP*. SAS Institute, Inc.

10

Monitoring Ambulance Diversion Hours

10.1 Key Concepts

Data visualization, descriptive statistics, control charts, common and special cause variation.

10.2 DMAIC

C: In this case, you will use tools that apply to the Control phase in the Define–Measure–Analyze–Improve–Control (DMAIC) process.

10.3 PDCA

C: In this case, you will use tools that apply to the Check step in the Plan–Do–Check–Act (PDCA) process.

10.4 Background

Cedars-Sinai Medical Center, located in Los Angeles, California, is an 886-bed nonprofit, academic medical center. The Cedars-Sinai Emergency Department is a Level 1 trauma center and has been designated as both a stroke and a ST-Elevation Myocardial Infarction (STEMI) receiving center. These designations mean that the emergency department (ED) is trained and equipped to treat patients with serious strokes and serious heart attacks that are characterized by complete blockage of one or more coronary arteries.

Improving Health Care Quality: Case Studies with JMP®, First Edition.
Mary Ann Shifflet, Cecilia Martinez, Jane Oppenlander, and Shirley Shmerling.
© 2020 John Wiley & Sons, Inc. Published 2020 by John Wiley & Sons, Inc.
Books Companion site:www.wiley.com/go/shifflet/improvinghealthcarequality1e

Ambulance diversion occurs when an ED sends ambulances to other facilities to help alleviate patient flow issues, such as ED overcrowding or when inpatient beds are not available. This practice has become common for hospitals in urban areas and for those that are trauma centers. As a result, patients can experience reduced quality of care and increased waiting times for treatment. The impact extends to the emergency medical services system by reducing the availability of ambulances and by increasing transport time and distances traveled. Hospitals suffer a loss of revenue from ambulance diversion.

Ambulance diversion is a nationwide problem, and many states have developed strategies to improve patient flow, both in the ED and throughout the hospital. Examples include reducing ED admission time through the use of kiosks, creating staff positions solely devoted to managing patient flow, and wirelessly transmitting electrocardiograms to the ED from the ambulance prior to patient arrival. The number of hours an ED is on ambulance diversion is a key performance measure for hospitals.

10.5   The Task

The objective of this case is to create control charts for Cedars-Sinai Medical Center to monitor the daily ambulance diversion hours.

10.6   The Data: CedarsSinai_Diversion_Hours.jmp

The California Health and Human Services Agency makes monthly hospital ambulance diversion data available to the public from their open data portal. The file CedarsSinai_Diversion_Hours.jmp contains simulated daily diversion hours for 2015, which we derived from the monthly values retrieved from the California Open Data Portal. The variables are defined in Table 10.1.

Table 10.1   Data definitions for Cedars-Sinai ambulance diversion.

Column name	Definition
Date	MM/DD/YYYY
Month	Month, e.g. January, February
Week	YYYY-WW
DOW	Day of the week, e.g. Monday, Tuesday
DiversionHrs	Total daily ambulance diversion hours

10.7   Data Management

The Date and Week columns were assigned a modeling type of continuous when imported into JMP® from the Excel file that was downloaded from the California Health and Human Services Open Data Portal. These two columns should be changed to an ordinal modeling type. To do this, double click on the column name to obtain the Column Information dialog. Change the modeling type to Ordinal from the dropdown menu. This is the only data processing needed.

10.8   Analysis

10.8.1   Descriptive Analysis

A run chart plots observations in time (or sequence) order. It is a good way to visualize time-dependent data, such as daily ambulance diversion, to become familiar with patterns of variation. Figure 10.1 shows the Cedars-Sinai daily ambulance diversion hours for 2015.

From this plot, we observe that there are a number of days where ambulance diversion did not occur and a noticeable dip in diversion hours from February to April.

Numerical statistics are also useful to quantify ambulance diversion hours. Figure 10.2 shows a histogram and descriptive statistics obtained from the

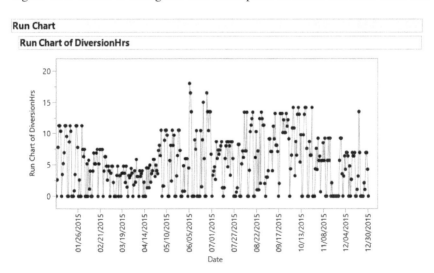

Figure 10.1   Run Chart for Cedars-Sinai ambulance diversion.
(Analyze > Quality and Process > Control Chart > Run Chart. Enter DiversionHrs in the Process field and Date in the Sample Label field.)

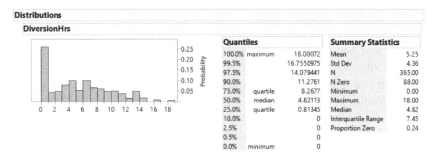

Figure 10.2   Distribution output for ambulance diversion hours. (Analyze > Distribution. Enter DiversionHrs in the Y, Columns field. Click OK. From the Summary Statistics dropdown menu select Customize Summary Statistics and choose the summary statistics shown.)

Distribution platform. The summary statistics have been rounded to two decimal places. (In the Summary Statistics table, double click over the column containing the numbers and choose the desired rounding from the resulting dialog.)

The mean daily ambulance diversion is 5.25 hours and the median is 4.82 hours. The variation as quantified by the standard deviation is 4.36 hours. The interquartile range, another measure of variation, is the range of the middle 50% (75th percentile to 25th percentile) of the data which is 7.45 hours. For 2015, 88 days (24%) did not experience ambulance diversion.

10.8.2   Control Chart Basics

Control charts are used to monitor a process to ensure that improvements are maintained over time. They allow the user to distinguish between common cause and special cause variation. The normal, expected fluctuations in a process measure are common cause variation. Unusual or unexpected fluctuations are special cause variation. Process owners take different approaches in response to common or special cause variation. Occurrences of special cause variation should be investigated and actions taken to remove the source of that variation. To reduce common cause variation, the system itself must be modified. Further detail on common and special cause variation can be found in Deming (1986).

There are a variety of different control charts. The appropriate chart to choose depends on the measurement level of the process variable being monitored. Control charts are categorized as either attribute charts that monitor defects or variables charts that monitor numeric process variables. Processes that are monitored with a numeric variable typically employ two control charts, one to track the process center and another to monitor variability. (See Chapter 11 for more information on control charts and Carey (2003) or Montgomery (2012).)

A control chart is a run chart, augmented with a center line and lower control limit (LCL) and upper control limit (UCL). The centerline and control limits are calculated from historical samples collected over time for a chosen statistic. The centerline is the average value of the statistic and the control limits define the region corresponding to common cause variation. The control limits are typically set at +/− three standard errors for the chosen statistic. The standard error is a measure of the variation in a sample statistic. For example, an X-bar chart monitors the process average where the center line is the average of the historical sample averages. The control limits are derived from the sample size and either the range, the standard deviation, or the moving range of the historical sample averages (Montgomery, 2012).

Once control charts are established, the process is monitored by periodically taking samples and plotting the values of the chosen statistic. Points falling within the control limits indicate that the process is stable and is operating as expected. Points falling outside of the control limits indicate the process has changed and investigation is needed to find and address the cause.

10.8.3 Ambulance Diversion Process

Ambulance diversion is an indicator of patient flow problems either in the ED or in other parts of the hospital. Many hospitals monitor the total number of hours an ED is on ambulance diversion status each day. Total ambulance diversion hours is a numeric measure and a pair of charts can be used to monitor the process center and variation. In this case, each day has only one value of total ambulance diversion hours, so the appropriate control charts to use are an I-chart (individual measurement) and an MR chart (moving range). The daily total ambulance diversion hours are plotted on the I-chart and the moving range is plotted on the MR chart. The moving range is an estimate of the variation and is calculated as the difference between the observation on one day and the observation on the previous day.

10.8.4 Setting the Control Limits

Before process monitoring can begin, the center lines and control limits must be established for the I and MR charts. Typically, about 25 to 30 historical observations are needed. Control limits should only be established when a process is stable. A run chart can be used to assess process stability. For this case, we will use the ambulance diversion hours from the month of November to establish the control limits. A JMP file containing just the November observations was created using Rows > Data Filter and then Tables > Subset. Figure 10.3 shows the run chart for November.

Run Chart

Run Chart of DiversionHrs

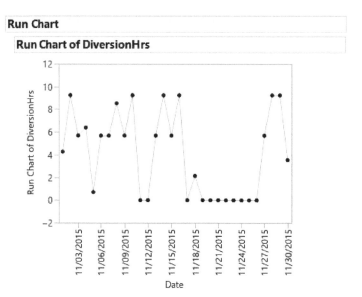

Figure 10.3   Run Chart for November Cedars-Sinai ambulance diversion. (Use Rows > Data Filter to select November data. Tables > Subset. Then follow the instructions from Figure 10.1.)

The run chart does not reveal any unusual observations that would be indicative of special cause variation that should be eliminated to achieve process stability. Figure 10.4 shows the I and MR charts created for the November ambulance diversion hours. JMP refers to the pair as "IR" charts.

Both the individual measurements and moving ranges for November are within the control limits. Diversion hours can never be negative, therefore, in this case, process outcomes will never be below the LCL in the I-chart. Once control limits are calculated, they are not changed as the ambulance diversion hours are added to the charts each day. Control limits can be saved in JMP either in a column in the active data table or in a new data table. For this case, we will save the control limits in a new data table named AmbulanceDiversion_ControlLimits.jmp. Select the dropdown menu from the Control Chart illustrated in Figure 10.4, choose Save Limits > in New Table. Figure 10.5 shows the data table containing the control chart information.

Now that the I- and MR-control charts are configured, monitoring can begin.

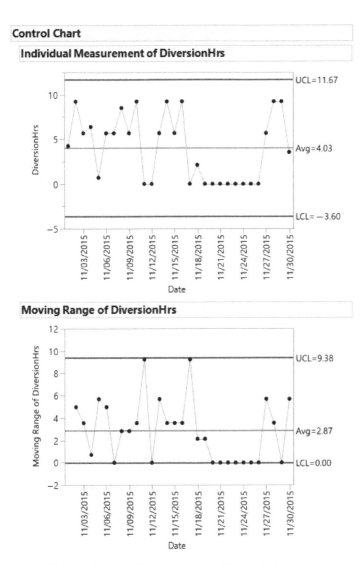

Figure 10.4 IR charts for November Cedars-Sinai ambulance diversion. (Analyze > Quality and Process > Control Chart > IR. Enter DiversionHrs in the Process field and Date in the Sample Label field. Check Individual Measurement and Moving Range(Average). Set Range Span to 2 and under Parameters set KSigma to 3. Click OK.)

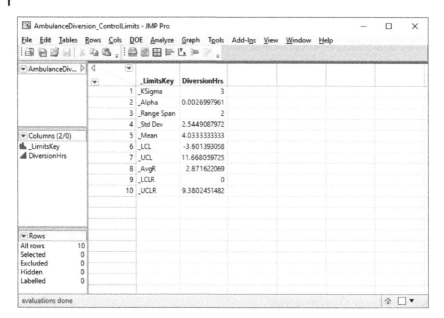

Figure 10.5 JMP data table with control chart values.

10.8.5 Monitoring Ambulance Diversion with IR Charts

In this case, since we are using historical data, the control limits calculated from the November ambulance diversion will be used to retrospectively assess the process performance for the 31 days of December. To begin, we will create a data table with just the December ambulance diversions and import the control limits from the file AmbulanceDiversion_ControlLimits.jmp. Return to the file CedarsSinai_Diversion_Hours.jmp and extract the subset of December ambulance diversion hours (Rows > Data Filter and then Tables > Subset). Figure 10.6 shows the control charts for the December ambulance diversion hours.

The ambulance diversion hours for 20 December (13.5 hours) exceed the upper control limit for both the I and MR charts. This indicates that both the process average and variation are considered out-of-control and the process owner should investigate to see what may have changed to cause this unusually high number of diversion hours and take appropriate corrective actions. In this case, we are looking at the data retrospectively. Control charts are a real time tool and in an actual application, at the end of each day the ambulance diversion hours would be plotted to determine if the process was out of control.

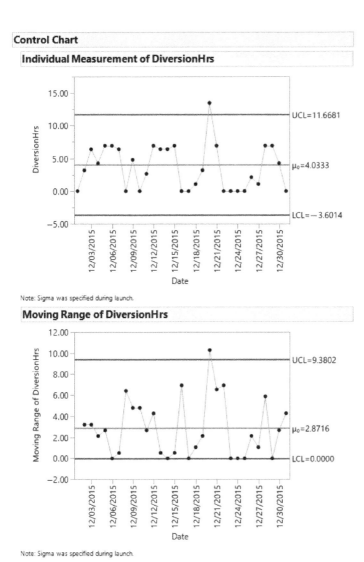

Figure 10.6 IR charts for December Cedars-Sinai ambulance diversion.
(Analyze > Quality and Process > Control Chart > IR. Enter DiversionHrs in the Process
field and Date in the Sample Label field. Click Get Limits and open the file
AmbulanceDiversion_ControlLimits.jmp. Click OK.)

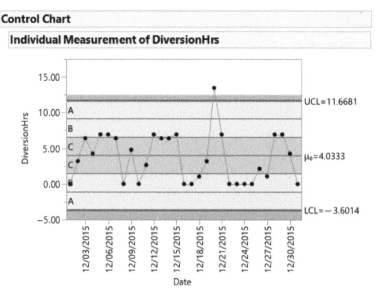

Note: Sigma was specified during launch.

Figure 10.7   I-chart for ambulance diversion with zones.
(From the Individual Measurements dropdown menu, select Show Zones and Shade Zones.)

In addition to using the control limits to signal when the process is out of control, there are sets of rules that can be applied to detect unusual patterns of variation that also indicate the process is out of control. JMP provides an option to use two sets of rules, the Western Electric rules and the Westgard rules. In this case, we will illustrate the Western Electric rules for the I-chart. The in-control region (inside of the control limits) of the I-chart is divided into zones. Zone C lies one standard error above and below the center line, Zone B lies from one standard error to two standard errors above and below the centerline, and Zone A lies from two standard errors above and below the centerline to the control limits. Figure 10.7 shows these zones for the I-chart.

There are eight Western Electric rules that can be applied to detect unusual patterns of variation. For example, Test 1 looks for one point that lies beyond Zone A (this is the case for the December 20th observation) and Test 6 looks for four out of five consecutive points in Zone B or beyond and the point itself lies in Zone B or beyond. The user may select to apply any or all of these tests.

Figure 10.8 shows the results of implementing all eight tests for the I-chart. Notice the annotation that Rule 1 has been violated on 20 December and Rule

Control Chart

Individual Measurement of DiversionHrs

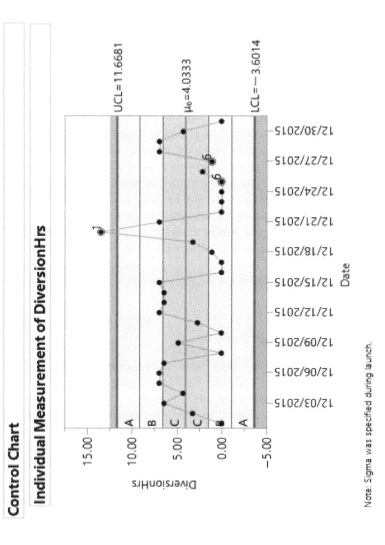

Figure 10.8 I-chart for ambulance diversion with zones and Western Electric rules. (From the Individual Measurements dropdown menu, select Tests > All Tests.)

6 has been violated on both 25 December and 27 December. After one of the Western Electric rules has been violated, the process owner should investigate to see what changes or special causes of variation have occurred and take appropriate corrective action. For additional description of the Western Electric and Westgard rules, see Help > Books > Quality and Process Methods (JMP 2018).

10.9 Summary

10.9.1 Statistical Insights

In the ambulance diversion case we found that control charts provide an objective means to establish levels of acceptable variation and identify variation that is attributable to special causes, signaling to the process owner when corrective actions are needed. Controls charts have proven to be effective tools for process monitoring and can be easily implemented by those workers who are directly involved with the process. This allows quick response to return the process to control and can limit the magnitude of the problem. Control charts differentiate between variation that is a natural part of the system and that which is unusual and should be addressed. Responding to variation that is within the natural (or common cause) variation can lead to "overcorrecting" the process which may result in wasted effort, additional system problems, and increased system variability.

10.9.2 Implications and Next Steps

Control charts allow stakeholders throughout an organization to monitor and visualize process performance. This helps maintain process improvements over time and signals when corrective actions are indicated.

In this case, IR charts were created and the process performance for a one month period was examined retrospectively. In practice, at the end of each day, the ambulance diversion hours for that day would be plotted on IR charts. Ambulance diversion is one example of a process measure that is used to monitor patient flow. Other performance measures, as appropriate to each organization, should be identified and monitored. However, only the "vital few"measures should be chosen. Monitoring requires resources and a minimum number of process characteristics should be tracked so that staff are not overburdened with this activity.

10.9.3 Summary of Tools and JMP Features

Statistical methods tools	Data management concepts	JMP platform features	Quality tools
Descriptive statistics	Data typing	Distribution	Common cause variation
			Special cause variation
Data visualization	Data filtering	Quality and process	
– *Histogram*			
– *Run chart*			
– *Control chart*			
Western Electric rules for control charts	Subsetting	Data filter	
		Tables > Subset	

10.9.4 Exercises

1. Repeat the analysis given in this case for Harbor-UCLA Medical Center, a 570-bed teaching hospital funded by the county of Los Angeles. The data can be found in the file HarborUCLA_Diversion_Hours.jmp. How do the results compare to those of the Cedars-Sinai Medical Center?
2. Experiment with different options for the Harbor-UCLA Medical control charts.
   (a) Try different combinations of the Western Electric rules (Tests) or the West-gard rules.
   (b) Try different visualization options, for example showing zones.
   (c) Create the Individual and Moving Range charts for this data that you think is best for this situation. Explain your choice of control chart options.
3. Create variability charts for the Cedars-Sinai Medical Center data (Analyze > Quality and Process > Variability/Attribute Gauge Chart) to visualize patterns

of variability in the ambulance diversion hours by month and week. Prepare a paragraph that summarizes your observations.

4. Using the Cedars-Sinai Medical Center data, recreate the control charts presented in this case using JMP's Control Chart Builder. Experiment with the different options and compare your results to those presented in this case.

5. Brainstorm possible causes of ambulance diversion. Create a cause-and-effect diagram using the JMP Diagram feature (Analyze > Quality and Process > Diagram). Use JMP documentation to learn how to create your diagram.

10.9.5 Discussion Questions

1. Search the Internet to find best practices for reducing ambulance diversion. Describe where these quality improvements occur in the patient flow process and how they reduce ambulance diversion.

2. The Donabedian model is a framework used for evaluating healthcare delivery and quality of patient care. The model describes three domains that affect healthcare quality: structure, process, and outcome. Find a reference that describes an application of the Donabedian model in emergency medical services. Prepare a brief summary of how the process is modeled.

3. Create a high-level process diagram of the US emergency medical services system. Identify key quality measures at each process step.

References

Carey, R.G. (2003). *Improving Healthcare With Control Charts: Basic and Advanced SPC Methods and Case Studies)*. ASQ.

Deming, W.E. (1986). *Out of the Crisis*, 2e. MIT Press.

JMP (2018). *Quality and Process Methods*. SAS Institute, Inc.

Montgomery, D.C. (2012). *Statistical Quality Control*, 7e. Wiley.

11

Ambulatory Surgery Start Times

11.1 Key Concepts

Statistical process control (SPC), control charts, common and special cause variation, stratification.

11.2 DMAIC

C: In this case, you will use tools that apply to the Control phase in the Define–Measure–Analyze–Improve–Control (DMAIC) process.

11.3 PDCA

CA: In this case, you will use tools that apply to the Check and Act steps in the Plan–Do–Check–Act (PDCA) process.

11.4 Background

Due to the unpredictability of surgical procedure durations, operating rooms (ORs) are difficult to schedule and are expensive areas in the hospital. One of the immediate consequences of OR inefficiencies is delayed surgeries. Starting surgeries after their scheduled time contributes to decreased OR utilization, leading to higher hospital costs, as well as reduced patient and hospital staff satisfaction. In this case, a rural hospital in upstate New York seeks to evaluate and improve their OR efficiency, which would allow this hospital to perform more surgeries for the same cost.

Improving Health Care Quality: Case Studies with JMP®, First Edition.
Mary Ann Shifflet, Cecilia Martinez, Jane Oppenlander, and Shirley Shmerling.
© 2020 John Wiley & Sons, Inc. Published 2020 by John Wiley & Sons, Inc.
Books Companion site:www.wiley.com/go/shifflet/improvinghealthcarequality1e

The hospital leadership was particularly interested in improving the performance of their ambulatory surgery unit (ASU). Their concern was that surgeries were starting much later than their scheduled times. Ambulatory surgeries could be scheduled in any of the four operating rooms from 7:30 a.m. to 5 p.m. any day of the week and were performed by the ASU staff and a team of 16 surgeons. The leadership team had the perception that delayed surgeries was a major problem for the first surgery scheduled in the day (referred to here as case 1 surgery) and not so much in the subsequent surgeries scheduled throughout the day (case 2 surgeries). They wanted to focus on case 1 surgeries since they typically play a critical role in setting the dynamics of how the OR will function throughout the remainder of the day. Although leadership was most concerned with case 1 surgeries, a task force team was assigned to assess the performance of both surgery cases. By looking at both cases, the task force believed they could better identify the areas that would warrant improvement efforts.

11.5 The Task

The task force chose to evaluate ASU surgery start time performance in two ways. One way was to consider whether the surgery was late or not, using both a 5-minute and a 15-minute threshold values for considering the surgery late. The other way was to look at the number of minutes late for the start of surgery. For either case, control charts were used to evaluate the processes.

11.6 The Data: ASU.jmp

The data set contains ambulatory surgical records from the last 13 weeks of 2017 from the top three surgeons in terms of the volume of surgical cases. These surgeons accounted for 44% of the total number of ASU surgeries in that time period. Both case 1 and case 2 surgeries are included. For purposes of this case, only a sample of the case 2 surgeries is included in this data set.

The variables in the data set are given in Table 11.1.

11.7 Data Management

The only data management needed is to create a new variable from the Late/On Time variable that is a yes/no variable: late, not late. To do this right, click on the Late/On Time variable column, select Recode, provide a new variable name (such as CategoryLate) and code Late as Late and both Early and On time as not late.

Table 11.1 Variable definitions.

Variable	Definition
Date	MM\DD\YYYY
Day	1 = Monday, 7 = Sunday
Week	1–52
Year	2017
Scheduled Start Time	
Case Variable	1 = first surgery of the day, 2 = subsequent surgeries
OR Room Scheduled	A, B, C, D
Case Start Time	
Late/On Time	Late, Early, On time
Late > 5 min	1 = late, 0 = not late
Late > 15 min	1 = late, 0 = not late
If Late, by how much	Number of minutes late – negative values indicate surgery started early
Case End	End time of surgery
Anes Type	Type of anesthesia
Surgeon Number	1, 3, and 7 – identifies specific surgeon
Procedure	Type of surgery
Incision	Time of first incision
Close	Time of surgery close

11.8 Analysis

SPC examines a process over time and uses process variable averages and variability to determine if the process operation is consistent, stable, or "in control." A consistent process signifies that the fluctuations observed in its performance are most likely due to common cause variation. Control charts are typically used to determine when special cause variation has occurred and corrections to the process need to be performed. Control limits are determined based on historical data from the process. Special cause variation is detected by values of the sample statistic outside of the control limits or a nonrandom pattern in the data such as those defined by the Westgard rules in JMP®.

SPC can be used for retrospective analysis or real-time process monitoring. In this case, the task force team wanted to use control charts for evaluating historical

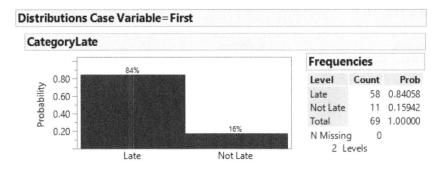

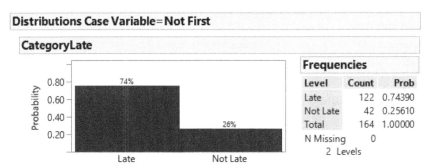

Figure 11.1   Distribution of late surgeries by type of case.
(Analyze > Distribution; Drag CategoryLate to Y, Columns box; drag Case Variable to By box. Click OK. Click on red triangle next to Distributions, select Stack.)

process performance. The team was interested in knowing to what extent ASU surgeries have been consistently meeting expectations for starting on time.

The team started the analysis by exploring the data collected. They first wanted to know the percentages of late surgeries for each case. Figure 11.1 shows the distribution of late surgeries for each case. Both types of surgeries, case 1 and case 2, have a high percentage of late surgeries, 84.1% for case 1 and 74.4% for case 2.

The next logical question for the task force team to answer was by how much have these surgeries been delayed? Figure 11.2 shows the dot plots of the difference between the actual and scheduled start times shown in minutes on the *y*-axis. There are six dot plots, stratified by case and surgeon. A quick inspection of the graph reveals that even though a higher percentage of case 1 surgeries are late, the number of minutes late is typically much lower than for the case 2 surgeries. Moreover, the variability is also much larger for the later surgeries than the ones scheduled in the first hour of the morning. Figure 11.3 provides the mean and standard deviations for each of these groups.

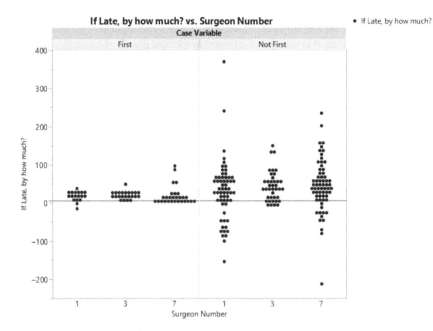

Figure 11.2 Dot plots of differences between scheduled and start of surgery times. (Graph > Graph Builder. Drag If Late, by how much? to *y*-axis; Drag Surgeon Number to *x*-axis; drag Case Variable to Group X area. Scroll over *y*-axis until hand tool appears, right click, add a reference line at 5.)

	If Late, by how much?					
	Case Variable					
	First			Not First		
	Surgeon Number			Surgeon Number		
	1	**3**	**7**	**1**	**3**	**7**
N	18.00	23.00	28.00	60.00	39.00	65.00
Mean	13.39	17.30	18.57	28.10	41.87	41.51
Std Dev	11.06	9.11	24.34	78.59	38.61	67.62
Min	−15.00	6.00	0.00	−154.00	−8.00	−212.00
Max	30.00	49.00	95.00	370.00	150.00	235.00

Figure 11.3 Summary statistics for If Late, by how much. (Analyze > Tabulate. Drag If Late, by how much? to the Drop Zone for columns; drag and drop Case Variable just below If Late, by how much?; drag and drop Surgeon Number just below Case Variable. Drag N, Mean, Std Dev, Min, and Max to Drop Zone for rows. Change the format to two decimal places by clicking on Change Format in the lower left corner; select Use the same decimal format; select Fixed Dec and select 2 decimal places.)

For both cases, there are a substantial number of dots (surgeries) above the reference line shown at five minutes. Given the number of surgeries exceeding the five-minute threshold, it is possible that the five-minute goal is not reasonable. In spite of this, all three surgeons have some surgeries starting earlier than the scheduled time with two of the surgeons (1 and 7) having a large number of surgeries starting early. For case 1 surgeries, it appears that surgeon 7 has several surgeries starting over 45 minutes late.

After looking at the overall process performance for the last three months the team decided to investigate the performance over time. Historical data from an inconsistent or unstable process cannot predict future process performance and is not suitable for process improvement efforts. The approach should be first to stabilize the process, that is, eliminate special cause variation, and once the process is in control, make the appropriate changes to bring it to the desired level of operation.

SPC allows the monitoring of process outputs that can be measured numerically or by attributes. The team first decided to create a series of control charts for numerical variables, that is, the surgery start time deviations from the scheduled times. However, the two groups of surgeries, case 1 and case 2, require different type of variable control charts that monitor both the target level of performance as well as its variability.

11.8.1 Case 1 Analysis

The chart for individuals (or I-charts) were used for depicting the process performance of all case 1 surgeries for the three-month period. Unlike the rest of the control charts that are based on sample statistics, the points plotted in I-charts are the individual observations of a given process performance characteristic. In this case, the team only had one surgery scheduled per operating room, that is a sample size of one. Charts for individuals are also used when the process for collecting the sample data takes too long or it is too expensive to conduct the measurement of the quality characteristic under study.

Figure 11.4 shows the pairs of individual and moving range (MR) charts for each surgeon for the case 1 surgeries. The center line is the overall average of the data points. The control limits are computed based on the MR, which is the absolute difference between two consecutive observations. When there is only one observation per time period, the MR is used as a measure of process variability. Note that the process for surgeon 7 exhibits much more variability than the other two surgeons. The process variability is reflected in the spread of the control limits for both charts, I- and MR-charts. The control limits of case 1 surgeries with the other two surgeons are narrower than the control limits of case 1 surgeries for surgeon 7.

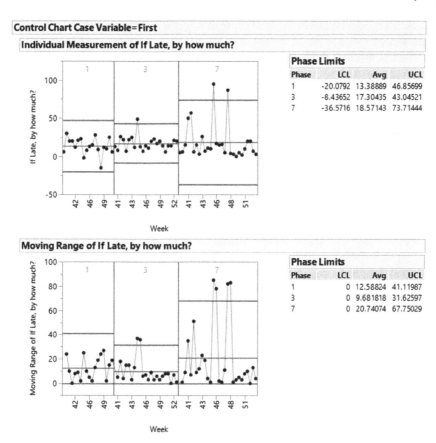

Figure 11.4 I-charts and MR-charts for case 1 surgeries.
(Sort the data by Case Variable and Surgeon Number by selecting Tables > Sort. Select Analyze > Quality and Process. Select Control Chart, select IR; Drag If Late, by how much? to the Process box; Drag Week to the Sample Label box; drag Surgeon Number to the Phase box; Drag Case Variable to By box. Click OK.)

Surgeons 3 and 7 have similar average numbers of minutes late, with 17.3 and 18.6 minutes, respectively. Surgeon 1 has a somewhat lower average of 13.4 minutes.

From the three sets of control charts in Figure 11.4, the control chart for case 1 surgeries performed by surgeon 1 did not show signs of instability. This process also has the closest actual average start times to the target time. That is, on average, the surgery starts 8.4 minutes past the five-minute tolerance. However, for the other two surgeons, there are data points that fall beyond the upper control limits, suggesting an "out-of-control" process. Even after conducting some investigations, the task force could not find special circumstances that could be linked to such large deviations in the start times of surgeon 7's first surgeries of weeks 45 and 48.

The task force also looked at historical records of case 1 surgeries from surgeon 3. The team wanted to identify a special cause that could explain the data point plotted beyond the upper control limit found in the I-chart at week 43, with a delay of 49 minutes. After looking at the hospital patient registration records, the task force team found that the patient arrived late to the hospital. Even though patient check-in times are beyond the hospital staff control, the team recommended an initiative for raising patient awareness of the importance of on-time check-in for their scheduled ambulatory surgeries and its impact on other patient surgeries.

One potential problem with the data points that lie beyond the control limits is that they inflate the variability and make the control limits wider than they should be. In practice, these data points are omitted from the control limit computations if these sample data points can be associated with a special-cause event and the appropriate corrective action has been implemented. However, this situation was not the case for the case 1 surgeries of surgeon 7 and raised concerns among the team members about the validity of these control limits.

Since the I- and MR-charts are sensitive to the assumption that the data is normally distributed, consideration should be given to whether the assumption is valid. A test such as the Shapiro–Wilk test can be used to check this assumption. If it is determined that the normality assumption is not valid then an Exponentially Weighted Moving Average (EWMA) chart may be more appropriate (see Exercise 7.) For more details on EWMA control charts see Montgomery (2012).

Overall, the control charts in Figure 11.4 indicate that the process of first case surgeries is not stable, making this process difficult to predict and improve. It appears that there are other process input variables or interactions besides the surgeon who performs the medical procedure. Further investigation is warranted to uncover the causes of the instability.

11.8.2 Case 2 Analysis

For the rest of the surgeries scheduled throughout the day, that is for case 2 surgeries, the task force decided to use a series of X-bar and range charts. These charts are appropriate for monitoring numeric variables where the sample size is 2 or greater. The X-bar chart is used to monitor the average of a process performance characteristic. The mean is important because it is an indicator of whether the process is operating at the desired target level. However, large and small values in a sample may produce an average value close to the target level when in reality the process produces outputs far from the desired target level. Therefore, the range chart complements the analysis by monitoring the performance variability, as measured by the difference between the highest and lowest values in a sample.

In SPC analysis, the objective is to use both charts to identify when a process should continue its operations and when investigations should be conducted. When creating a control chart, small samples, typically 2–10, are taken at regular time intervals to ascertain the process performance. These are referred to as rational subgroups and are a measure of process performance at a snapshot in time. Based on the volume of surgeries performed, rational subgroup sizes of five per week were chosen for surgeons 1 and 7, and three per week for surgeon 3. Figure 11.5 shows the X-bar and R charts for each surgeon for the case 2 surgeries. The charts reveal that the start time performance of case 2 surgeries is not in control, regardless of the surgeon. For two of the surgeons, 1 and 7, the control limit widths of the range charts are very similar (about 254 minutes), as are the average ranges, with both being about 120 minutes. Surgeon 3 has a much lower average range (48 minutes) than the other two surgeons. Both surgeons 1 and 7 have observations outside the control limits of the range charts, suggesting unstable variability. Surgeon 1 has a lower average number of minutes late than the other two surgeons. Notice, also, that three of the "out of control" points for surgeon 1 are on the low side and, in fact, are negative, indicating that the average start times for his surgeries for that week were actually earlier than scheduled. The variability in average minutes late is the smallest for surgeon 3 as seen in the narrower control limits. The team would need to follow up with the three surgeons to determine why surgeon 1 was able to have earlier than scheduled start times and why surgeon 3 had less variability. Uncovering these special causes could allow for more standardization in procedures and efficiency in the ASU.

After sharing the process assessment results with the surgeons and leadership team, one particular surgeon showed genuine commitment to improving the performance of his surgery start times. By streamlining communication and patient awareness, the process started to run more consistently. Table 11.2 shows data collected for surgeon 1 in weeks 18–20 of 2018. The means are well inside the 2017 X-bar control limits and the ranges for weeks 18 and 19 are well below the 2017 average range. These results are encouraging, prompting the surgical staff to focus on maintaining good patient communication and inspiring the task force to search for additional opportunities to improve efficiency and reduce surgery start delays.

11.9 Summary

11.9.1 Statistical Insights

SPC is a key element in process improvement. The first step in SPC is to have clearly defined performance metrics. At the outset of this case, performance goals and metrics were unclear. The team chose to use both numeric (number of minutes late) and categorical (proportion late) to evaluate the process performance.

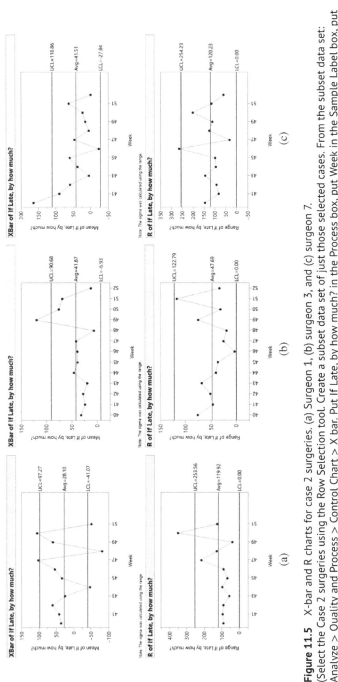

Figure 11.5 X-bar and R charts for case 2 surgeries. (a) Surgeon 1, (b) surgeon 3, and (c) surgeon 7. (Select the Case 2 surgeries using the Row Selection tool. Create a subset data set of just those selected cases. From the subset data set: Analyze > Quality and Process > Control Chart > X bar. Put If Late, by how much? in the Process box, put Week in the Sample Label box, put Surgeon Number in the By box. Click on Sample Size Constant and input 5 in the box. Click OK. This will provide the charts for surgeons 1 and 7. Redo the analysis with Sample Size Constant equal to 3 to obtain the correct charts for surgeon 3.)

Table 11.2 2018 data for surgeon 1.

Week	*n*	Mean	Standard deviation	Range
18	5	39.6	7.8	20
19	5	−15.0	22.33	55
20	1	59.0		

Typically, goals are based on past history, benchmarking, or industry best practice and in this case, the hospital leadership may have established goals that were unrealistic based on the variability in the system. Unrealistic goals can lead to demoralizing staff, rather than improving the process.

The control charts were used to assess historical data. The charts showed an unstable or inconsistent process. This was not a surprise to the hospital staff as they had been dealing with a process that runs differently depending on the surgery case and surgeon. This emphasizes the importance of understanding controllable and uncontrollable factors. The staff was surprised, however, to find a large number of delays during the first case of the day. No justification could be found for these delays. The ORs were left ready the night before and patients typically checked in on time. However, the hospital staff was not aware of the performance of the process and thus the control charts uncovered an issue that could be investigated. The use of data can also help in moving away from assigning misguided or anecdotal causes for OR delays, which in the end do nothing to either stabilize or improve the process performance. The analysis that this task force team conducted helped in increasing personal accountability, initiating projects for streamlining of procedures, promoting interdisciplinary teamwork, and defining mechanisms for accurate data collection. All of these aspects are an important part of process improvement.

11.9.2 Implications and Next Steps

This analysis was used to highlight the problem of late surgeries in the ASU. Prior to this project, this metric was not monitored at all, and the hospital staff and surgeons were unaware of their performance. Further investigation was required to map the process and identify causes of late surgeries to improve efficiency in this department. The major recommendation was to standardize processes across surgeons. This standardization led to improved efficiency and ultimately to achieving the targeted performance level. A secondary recommendation was to continue monitoring the process and make it available to the hospital staff so that the improvements would be maintained.

11.9.3 Summary of Tools and JMP Features

Statistical methods tools	Data management concepts	JMP platform features	Quality tools
Data visualization	Derived data	Tabulate	Process variation
– Dot plot			
– I-chart			
– MR-chart			
– X-bar chart			
– Range chart			
– p-Chart (Exercises 2–4)			
– EWMA chart (Exercise 7)			
Descriptive statistics		Distribution	Sources of variation
Normality test		Graph builder	Stratification
Control charts		Quality and process	Control charts
		Formula editor	

11.9.4 Exercises

1. Use JMP to get a basic statistical summary for each subgroup of data for the number of surgery start time delays.
   (a) By surgeon.
   (b) By surgery case.
   (c) By surgeon and surgery case.
2. The file LateSurgeries_ControlChart.jmp contains the number of weekly surgeries and the number of those surgeries that were late by 5 and 15 minutes.
   (a) Does this data represent defects or defectives? Explain the difference. (*Hint*: See Section 1.5.3.)
   (b) What is the appropriate type of control chart to monitor the late surgeries? (Hint: See Figure 11.4.) Explain why you chose this type of chart.
   (c) Construct two control charts, one for the surgeries that were more than five minutes late and one for the surgeries that were more than 15 minutes late.
   (d) Describe the appearance of the control limits on your charts and give an explanation based on your statistical knowledge.
   (e) Write a brief summary (two to three sentences) explaining the performance of the process using the 5-minute and the 15-minute thresholds.

3. Create the set of p-charts for case 2 surgeries. Use the five-minute threshold value to determine late surgeries. Get one p-chart for each surgeon. What can be said about the process performance? Is it in control? Discuss.
4. Use the appropriate statistical tool to test if there is a statistical difference in the variability across surgeons for each surgery case and between surgery cases.
5. Assume that the task force identified a special cause event for all the points that are plotted beyond the control limits from Figure 11.4 and that a corrective action was implemented. Reconstruct the control charts by omitting these out-of-control data points in the computations of the control limits. Is the process now in control? Are there points that plot beyond the new control limits? Discuss.
6. Repeat Exercise 5 for the X-bar and R charts given in Figure 11.5.
7. For the case 1 surgeries conduct a Shapiro–Wilk test of normality for each doctor. For the doctors whose data does not follow a normal distribution create an EWMA control chart. Discuss how an EWMA chart differs from an I-MR chart and summarize your conclusions.

11.9.5 Discussion Questions

1. There is a close connection between hypothesis testing and control charts. Discuss the similarities and differences.
2. A stable process or a process that is in control is not necessarily a good process. Explain why or why not.
3. Discuss the advantages and disadvantages of using control charts for variables and for attributes. When is it more convenient to use variables vs. attributes and vice versa?
4. Discuss other scenarios in which the charts of individual observations are useful.
5. Discuss what consequences would be seen in a process if small changes are made to the process every time the control chart triggers the signal of a potential out-of-control situation. Would these changes help reduce variability? Discuss.

Reference

Montgomery, D.C. (2012). *Statistical Quality Control*, 7e. Wiley.

12

Pre-Op TJR Process Improvement – Part 1

12.1   Key Concepts

Problem definition, exploratory analysis, stratification.

12.2   DMAIC

D: The tools illustrated in this case are frequently applied in the Define phase of the Define–Measure–Analyze–Improve–Control (DMAIC) approach to process improvement.

12.3   PDCA

PC: The tools illustrated in this case are frequently applied in the Plan and Check steps of the Plan–Do–Check–Act (PDCA) approach to process improvement.

12.4   Background

Patients requiring a total joint replacement (TJR) need to complete a preoperative process that includes surgery scheduling, primary care provider (PCP) clearance for surgery, preadmission testing, and patient education intended to help them adjust to their new lifestyle with a prosthetic. In a rural hospital in Upstate New York, the preoperative TJR process took longer than expected about 50% of the time. In this and the next two chapters, we show how the hospital, that was

Improving Health Care Quality: Case Studies with JMP®, First Edition.
Mary Ann Shifflet, Cecilia Martinez, Jane Oppenlander, and Shirley Shmerling.
© 2020 John Wiley & Sons, Inc. Published 2020 by John Wiley & Sons, Inc.
Books Companion site:www.wiley.com/go/shifflet/improvinghealthcarequality1e

struggling to consistently get patients through the preoperative TJR process without delays or rescheduled appointments, streamlined the process, and reduced avoidable delays and process variability through data analysis.

The measure of success or primary metric is the preoperative TJR process elapsed time, that is, the time in days that it takes for patients to complete the preoperative process. This process starts when the patient meets with the orthopedic doctor. In this visit, all medical appointments are scheduled in preparation for the TJR surgery. Figure 12.1 depicts a high-level process map of the preoperative TJR case. For each process step, the inputs and respective suppliers were identified as well as the outputs and customers for each output. This type of process map is known as a SIPOC diagram, which stands for suppliers, inputs, process, outputs, and customers. Among the people involved in this process are the patient receiving the knee or hip implant, the clinic scheduler, the PCP, the lab specialists, the operating room (OR) scheduler, internal and external labs, preadmission nurses, and the orthopedic doctors.

SIPOC diagrams such as the one shown in Figure 12.1 are useful for identifying and displaying the major steps of a process under study. Typically, these high-level process maps allow identification of upstream activities that may be causing undesirable outcomes downstream in the process, allowing teams to narrow the scope of the project.

12.5   The Task

Explore historical data to define and understand the problem, scope the project, and set project goals accordingly. It is unclear if the process improvement team should focus on the preoperative process of both knee and hip replacements or only one of them.

12.6   The Data: TJR.xlsx

The data set contains the dates of all required medical appointments and approvals that the patient needs to complete prior to surgery. Among the dates collected are the first consultation/scheduler meeting dates, surgery dates, PCP appointment dates, and date preoperative clearance is received. Another important metric to monitor is the number of surgeries rescheduled. The file TJR.xlsx contains the appointment records of patients who went through the TJR preoperative process in late 2016 and early 2017. All personally identifiable information has been removed to protect patient privacy. The data set also contains variables that characterize each patient's preoperative process regarding the type of prosthetic, provider,

Suppliers	Inputs	Process	Output	Customer
Patient or Primary care provider	Need for joint examination Patient Orthopedic doctor	**1** Meet with orthopedic doctor	Operation room consent form Patient knowledge Surgery decision	Patient Scheduler
Orthopedic doctor	Orthopedic doctor's surgery decision Patient Scheduler	**2** Book preoperative appointments with scheduler	Primary care provider appointment Specialist appointment Patient booking sheet Preop booking sheet created	Primary care provider Patient Specialist Operation room scheduler
Patient Primary care provider	Patient Primary care provider	**3** Meet with primary care provider (within 30 days of surgery)	Patient clearance Prescriptions for lab work Specialist clearance	Scheduler Specialist Internal/External lab
Patient	Preadmission nurses Patient clearance Specialist clearance	**4** Go to the preoperation appointment	Swab tests Patient knowledge Preop letter Final clearance	Preadmission nurses Patient Orthopedic doctor

Figure 12.1 SIPOC diagram for the preoperative TJR process.

reason for visit, insurance company, whether the patient attended joint replacement training, whether the PCP is a network or out-of-network provider, and if the surgery was rescheduled or not. Table 12.1 presents the definition of all the variables found in the TJR.xlsx file.

12.7 Data Management

To prepare the TJR data for analysis, we begin by importing TJR.xlsx into JMP®. Figure 12.2 shows the Excel Import Wizard which allows the user to select the worksheets to import and identify the location and number of column headers.

The file will now open as a JMP data table. JMP allows a wide variety of file types to be imported (see filename dropdown menu). When importing from other (non.jmp) file formats, it is important to review the JMP columns to be sure the data and modeling types are as needed for the analysis.

Date/time variables often require reformatting once imported into JMP as is the case with the Date of Surgery, Date Scheduler Meeting, and a number of other columns in this data table. The Date of Surgery column imported as a character data type and a nominal modeling type. These will need to be changed to a numeric data type and an ordinal modeling type in order to plot by date and to perform date calculations. Right click the column heading for Date of Surgery and select Column Info from the menu. Change the Data Type to Numeric, from the Modeling Type dropdown choose Ordinal, and from the Format dropdown select Date > m/d/y. All other date columns are formatted similarly.

The final diagnosis (column Final Drg) was imported into JMP as a continuous modeling type which is not appropriate since this is a three digit numeric code for the diagnosis-related group. This should be changed to a nominal modeling type. Right click the column heading Final Drg and change the modeling type to Nominal.

Notice that there are 104 rows in the data table, but only 47 rows contain data. This can happen on occasion when importing from Excel files. Once verified that 47 is the correct number of observations, the unneeded rows can be safely deleted. Save the JMP data table as TJR.jmp.

Later in this case, the surgery dates will need to be analyzed by month; the existing data table gives surgery date in m/d/y format. To create a new column containing only the month of surgery, JMP's formula editor and date functions can be employed. The new column will be named Month (Date of surgery). Figure 12.3 shows the completed formula needed for the new column.

The Month function returns the month in numeric format (e.g., 10, 11, 12). The modeling type should be set to ordinal (right click the modeling type icon to the left of the Month (Date of surgery) and select Ordinal from the dropdown menu). JMP

Table 12.1 Variable definitions.

Variable	Definition
Age	Patient age (years)
ReasonforVisit	Primary diagnosis
Type of Surgery	Hip or knee
Joint Supplier	Name of prosthetic manufacturer
Surgery–Supplier–Provider	Type of surgery, manufacturer, surgeon
Date of Surgery	mm\dd\yy
FinalDrg	Diagnosis related group
Dx1Name	Primary diagnosis
Insurance	Name of patient's insurance company
Provider Code	Surgeon identifier
Provider	Surgeon
Date scheduler meeting	mm\dd\yy, first time visit to ortho clinic
Days Between Scheduler Meeting and Pre-op appt	Elapsed time in business days between first visit to ortho clinic and preoperative appt with the primary care provider
PCP Pre-op appt	mm\dd\yy, primary care provider preop appt
Days Between Pre-op appt and Pre-op clearance	Elapsed time in business days between appt with primary care provider and preoperative clearance received
Pre-op Clearance Received	mm\dd\yy
Days between Pre-op Clearance and Surgery	Elapsed time in business days between preop clearance and surgery date
Total Elapsed Business Days	Elapsed time in business days between first visit to ortho clinic and surgery date
PCP in-network?	Yes – in-network, no – out of network
Reschedule?	Yes – surgery date rescheduled, no – otherwise
Attended Joint Class	Yes – attended class, no – otherwise
Date of Joint Class	mm\dd\yy, date patient attended class
Days from consultation to joint class	Elapsed time in business days between first visit to ortho clinic and joint class
Days from joint class to PCP appt	Elapsed time in business days between appt with PCP and joint class
Nonworking Holidays 2016	Holiday dates included in preoperative process for particular case

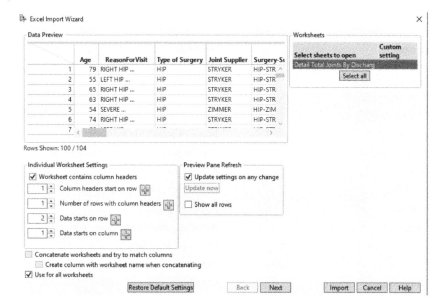

Figure 12.2 JMP Excel Import Wizard.
(File > Open. Select Excel Files (*.xls, *.xlsx, *.xlsm) from the filename dropdown menu.
Select TJR.xlsx and click Open. Click Import.)

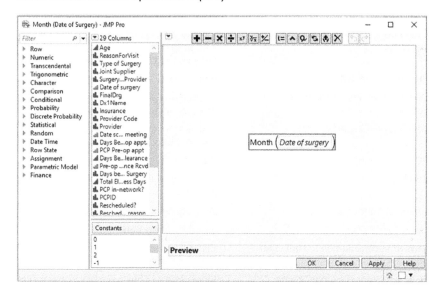

Figure 12.3 Formula editor to create Month (Date of Surgery).
(Select the Date column. Columns > New Column. Enter "Month (Date of surgery)" in the
Column Name field. Select Formula from the Column Properties dropdown, then click Edit
Formula. From the function list, select Date Time > Month. Click "Date of surgery" to
populate the formula. Click Apply. Click OK.)

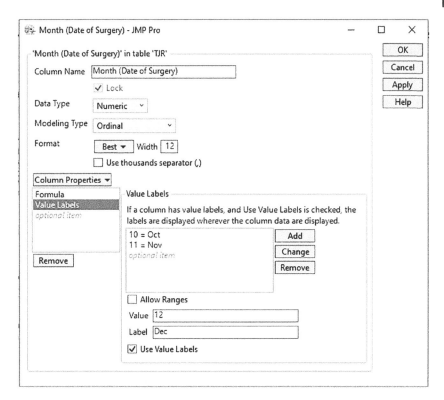

Figure 12.4 Setting Value Labels for Month (Date of Surgery).
(Right click column header for "Month (Date of surgery)" and select Column Info. Select Value Labels from the Column Properties dropdown menu. Enter each numeric month in the Value field and the desired character designation in the Label field. Click Add. Check Use Value Labels. Click Apply. Click OK.)

Value Labels can be set to cause the numeric month to be displayed as a character designation as shown in Figure 12.4. The three letter month abbreviation will be displayed in all subsequent output containing Month (Date of surgery).

12.8 Analysis

In defining the problem, we need to understand the performance baseline of the preoperative TJR process. We will use the data to answer questions such as how long does it typically take the patient to get to the operating room? One of the graphical tools that helps us see process behavior over time is the run chart (or time series plot). Figure 12.5 shows a run chart for the total elapsed days of the

Run Chart

Run Chart of Total Elapsed Business Days

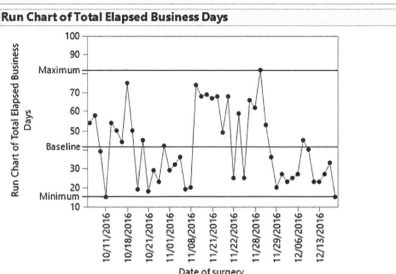

Figure 12.5   Run chart of elapsed time of the preop TJR process. (Analyze > Quality and Process > Control Chart > Run Chart. Select "Total Elapsed Business Days" and click "Process." Select "Date of Surgery" and click "Sample Label." For Sample Size, select "Sample Size Constant" and enter "1." Click "OK." To add reference lines to the chart: Right click on any value on the *y*-axis > Axis Settings. In Reference Lines: For Value enter 15. In Label, enter "Minimum." Click Add. Repeat to create a reference line for the maximum at 82 and baseline (average) at 41.5. (Note: reference values were obtained from Analyze > Distribution.)

preoperative TJR process. Notice that this graph has three added reference lines at the minimum, maximum, and average (labeled Baseline) values. These descriptive statistics were previously obtained from the Distribution platform. From this run chart, we identified that the total elapsed time (in business days) can be as little as 15 business days (three calendar weeks) or as long as 82 days (almost 17 weeks)!

A follow-up question is, why does this preoperative TJR process elapsed time have so much variability? We do not know if the problem lies in one step of the preoperative TJR process or if the inconsistent performance occurs throughout the entire process. This calls for a closer look at the process to obtain a better understanding of the current state, so the project team interviewed people involved in the process and obtained their insights. The project team learned that this preoperative process is very complex with the patient, doctor, scheduler, PCP, hospital and other lab personnel, preadmission testing nursing staff, and joint representatives all involved.

The preoperative TJR process starts when the patient meets with the orthopedic doctor who recommends a joint replacement. In this initial consultation, the patient also meets with the scheduler who sets appointments with the PCP and other specialists (if necessary), the joint class and the preadmission testing are also scheduled at this point. Once the scheduler verifies the insurance information and type of joint implant, she contacts the joint supplier and books a radiology appointment if the orthopedic surgeon has recommended the patient receive a Conformis knee replacement. Meanwhile, the patient is expected to attend the joint class and meet with the PCP no more than 30 days prior to surgery. The PCP decides whether additional testing is required for the patient. If no other testing is needed, the PCP sends its approval to the orthopedic clinic scheduler, which is recorded as the preoperative clearance received in the dataset. Then follows appropriate lab-work, ordering of prescriptions prior to surgery, and lastly, the swab test which has to be done no more than five days prior to surgery. Once all these requirements are met, the patient is ready for surgery.

With a better understanding of the process, the project team proceeded to identify stratification factors, which are factors that can be used to separate data into subgroups. Our objective is to identify where we should focus our improvement efforts. With the aid of a pie chart (Figure 12.6), we can look at the data by type

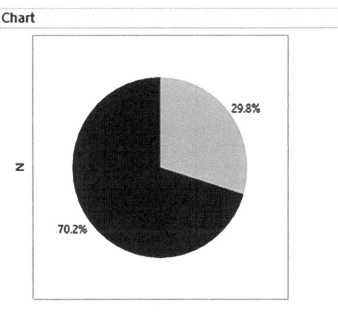

Figure 12.6 Pie chart of type of TJR surgery.
(Graph > Legacy > Chart. Select "Type of Surgery" and click Categories, X, Levels. Under Options select Pie chart (instead of Bar chart). Click OK. Right clicking anywhere on the pie will make a menu appear. In this menu, select Label > Label by percent of total value.)

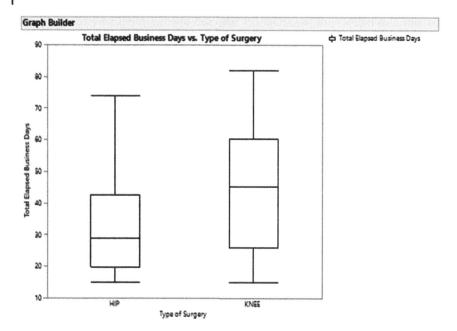

Figure 12.7 Summary statistics for If Late, by how much.
(Graph > Graph Builder. Drag Type of Surgery to x-axis; drag Total Elapsed Business Days
to y-axis; click on box plot icon at the top; click "Done.")

of implant. We see that 70% of the surgeries are related to knee implants, whereas
30% are hip surgeries.

We need to know which of the two preoperative processes takes the longest and
which one has more variation. Box plots help us visualize the center and the variability of a process. In looking at Figure 12.7, we see that the knee preoperative
process exhibits more variability and longer median elapsed time.

We can also visualize how long the process takes on average with a bar chart as
shown in Figure 12.8. To create this graph, we stratified the data by type of surgery,
month, and took the average times of the preop process of all patients who had
surgery in that given month. This bar chart suggests that the knee preoperative
process typically takes longer than the hip preoperative process.

We can further partition the data by the three process segments. The first segment is the elapsed days between the first consultation (meeting with the scheduler) and the appointment with the PCP. The second segment counts the elapsed

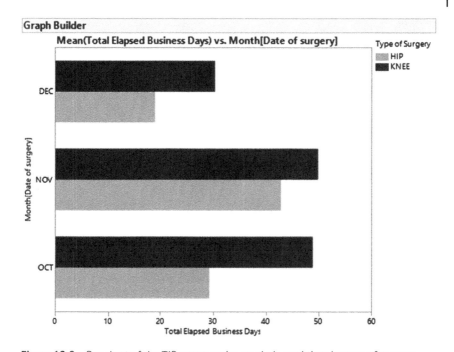

Figure 12.8 Bar chart of the TJR preoperative total elapsed time by type of surgery (business days).
(Graph > Graph Builder. Drag Total Elapsed Business Days to x-axis. Drag Month [Date of Surgery] to y-axis. Drag Total Elapsed Business Days to x-axis. Drag Type of Surgery to Overlay (on the right top of the panel); click on bars plot icon at the top.)

days between PCP appointment and the preoperative clearance. The last segment counts the elapsed days from the preoperative clearance and the surgery date. Figure 12.9 shows the bar chart, created in Graph Builder of the average times by process segment. From this stacked bar chart by process segments, it is evident that the largest average elapsed time occurs at the front-end of the preoperative process regardless of the type of implant. We can also observe that the third segment is longer for the knee preoperative process than for the hip preoperative process. Although stacked bar charts may not be considered best practice, in this case stacking the bars is helpful as it illustrates the chronology of the main process steps in a way that is easy to make comparisons. (See Exercise 4 for more discussion on stacked vs. nonstacked bar graphs.)

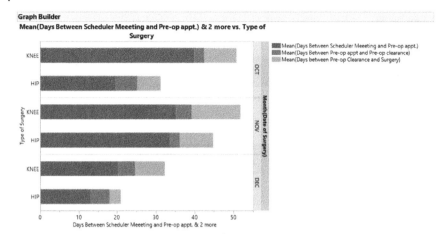

Figure 12.9 Bar chart of the average times of the TJR pre-op process elapsed times. (Graph > Graph Builder. Multiple select: "Days between Scheduler Meeting and Pre-op appt," "Days Between Pre-op appt and Pre-op Clearance" and "Days between Pre-op Clearance and Surgery." Drag the three selected columns to the x-axis. Drag "Type of Surgery" to the y-axis. Drag Month[Date of Surgery] to Group Y drop zone, and click the bar chart icon at the top. In Bar Style select "Stacked.")

The knee implants are higher in volume and its preoperative process takes longer and has greater variability. For these reasons, the process improvement team focused on the knee implants only. With this in mind, the team created another run chart for the knee implant data only. To obtain only the knee implant patients, create a filter for Type of Surgery by invoking Rows > Data Filter. Then, select "knee" and check "Show" and "Include" and then re-run the run chart. The result is the run chart shown in Figure 12.10 which shows with reference lines the best, baseline, and worst performances as well as the project goal set by leadership at 24 business days.

To better understand the knee preoperative process, the project team further sliced the data by type of knee implant. We are interested in determining if we should keep this stratification variable for further analysis. Another box plot was created where the stratification variables are the joint supplier and month. Figure 12.11 reveals that the preoperative process exhibits greater variability with the Conformis knee implant than with the Zimmer implant.

When we broke down the process as depicted in Figure 12.12, we noticed that the greatest part of the variability stems from the first day of consultation and the PCP appointment for the months of October and November. Interestingly, this was

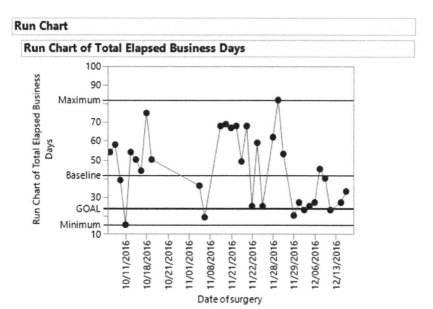

Figure 12.10 Run chart of the TJR preop elapsed time for knee implants only. (Analyze > Quality and Process > Control Chart > Run Chart. Select "Total Elapsed Business Days" and click "Process." Select "Date of Surgery" and click "Sample Label." For Sample Size, select "Sample Size Constant" and enter "1." Click "OK." Then, add Reference lines (minimum at 15, Goal at 24, Baseline at 41.5 and Maximum at 82).)

not the case for the month of December and warrants further investigation which will be considered for the next stages of the DMAIC.

12.9 Summary

12.9.1 Statistical Insights

In this first part of the case, we used historical data to conduct an exploratory analysis with the purpose of visualizing the performance of the preoperative TJR process. Data visualization tools are powerful for investigating process performance that can be easily assimilated by stakeholders with varying backgrounds. In the exploratory analysis, we used graphs such as run charts to see the process behavior over time; pie charts to determine the percentages of types of surgeries;

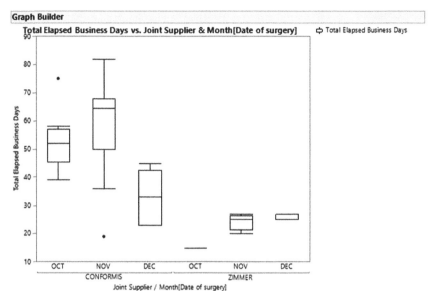

Figure 12.11   Box plot of total elapsed time for the knee pre-op process (business days). (Graph > Graph Builder. Then, drag Total Elapsed Business Days to *y*-axis. Next, drag Month[Date of Surgery] and "Joint Supplier" to the *x*-axis. Last, click on box plot icon at the top. Click "Done.")

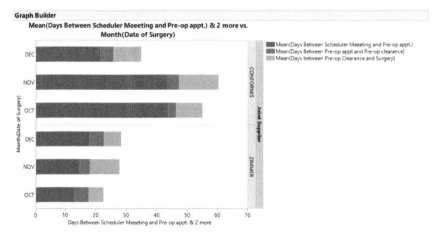

Figure 12.12   Bar chart of the average times for knee pre-op process elapsed times. (Graph > Graph Builder. Multiple select the variables: "Days between Scheduler Meeting and Pre-op appt," "Days Between Pre-op appt and Preop Clearance" and "Days between Preop Clearance and Surgery." Drag the three selected columns to *x*-axis. Then, drag Month[Date of Surgery] and "Joint Supplier" to *y*-axis. Last, click on bars plot icon at the top. In Bar Style select "Stacked.")

bar charts to determine the expected elapsed times of the process overall and by segments; and box plots to visualize the process variability. These visualizations helped the team understand the process performance and enabled them to narrow the scope of the problem. Defining the scope and goals of a process improvement project that align with the resources available are key to achieving success. Examining process performance by the various stratification factors (type of implant, month, and joint supplier) is crucial in project scoping. This allowed them to identify that more of the overall preoperative process variability comes from the Conformis knee implant and that the greatest source of variability appears in the early stages of the process, more specifically between the first consultation and the PCP appointment.

12.9.2 Implications and Next Steps

In Chapter 13, we will measure in a more detailed manner, the process capability, and calculate more descriptive statistics with the ultimate goal of identifying the critical factors that affect the overall process variability.

12.9.3 Summary of Tools and JMP Features

Statistical methods tools	Data management concepts	JMP platform features	Quality tools
Data visualization	Subsetting	Data filter	Process variation
– *Run chart*			
– *Pie chart*			
– *Bar chart*			
– *Box plot*			
Descriptive statistics	De-identification	Distribution	Sources of variation
	Derived data	Graph builder	Stratification
		Quality and process	Project scoping
		Formula editor	

12.9.4 Exercises

1. Use the file TJR.jmp to create a pie chart of the type of insurance. What is the most common insurance company? What would you do if the chart showed many "thin" slices?

2. Repeat Exercise 1. But this time, group the categories that have a frequency of less than 2.5%. Compare this new pie chart with the one created in Exercise 1. Which one do you think is better? Explain.

3. Create a run chart similar to Figure 12.10 with the reference lines for the baseline (average time), minimum, and maximum values but for the hip replacements only.

4. Consider the data used to create the bar charts shown in Figures 12.9 and 12.12 and create a side-by-side vertical bar chart. Compare and discuss the differences in displaying the same data. Which graph would be preferred? Why?

5. Use the file TJR.jmp to create a box plot of the patient ages. Use the same stratification by type of surgery as in Figures 12.6 and 12.7.

6. In this case, Value Labels were used to change the values of a variable displayed in JMP output. Explore other JMP methods that can be used to change how values are displayed (*Hint*: Cols > Recode). Compare and contrast the methods you discover with Value Labels.

12.9.5 Discussion Questions

1. Discuss why project scoping is critical for the success of a project.

2. Explain what a stratification factor is and the role it plays in project scoping. Find examples in the healthcare quality literature.

3. Discuss the difference in the graphical tools used for project scoping (run charts, box plots, bar charts, and pie charts.) When is one graph more appropriate to use than another?

4. When creating a bar chart, it is generally preferred (Tufte, 2001) to have side-by-side bars rather than stacked bars. It is also more common to see vertical bars than horizontal bars. However, Figures 12.9 and 12.12 show stacked and horizontal bars. Discuss what advantages (if any) a stacked, horizontal bar would have over a side-by-side vertical bar chart.

5. Discuss in what other ways the analysis of a distribution can be done in JMP. Which one do you prefer and why?

6. Discuss the different ways color can be used in graphs and investigate the pros and cons that these ways of using color can have on graph visualization.

7. In addition to color, the way data is separated or sliced affects the graph visualization making it harder or easier to understand. Discuss when it is more convenient to create a graph in separate panels vs. overlaid.

Reference

Tufte, E.R. (2001). *The Visual Display of Quantitative Information*, 2e. Graphics Press.

13

Pre-Op TJR Process Improvement – Part 2

13.1 Key Concepts

Exploratory analysis, coefficient of variation (CV), process capability analysis, variation.

13.2 DMAIC

MA: The tools illustrated in this case are frequently applied in the Measure and Analyze phases of the Define–Measure–Analyze–Improve–Control (DMAIC) approach to process improvement.

13.3 PDCA

PC: The tools illustrated in this case are frequently applied in the Plan and Check steps of the Plan–Do–Check–Act (PDCA) approach to process improvement.

13.4 Background

In Chapter 12, the use of exploratory data analysis, primarily through data visualization, illustrated how a process improvement team examined the performance of the total joint replacement (TJR) process to narrow the scope of the project. They found that focusing on the preoperative process for knee replacements only, would have the best potential for process improvement. The goal is to decrease

Improving Health Care Quality: Case Studies with JMP®, First Edition.
Mary Ann Shifflet, Cecilia Martinez, Jane Oppenlander, and Shirley Shmerling.
© 2020 John Wiley & Sons, Inc. Published 2020 by John Wiley & Sons, Inc.
Books Companion site:www.wiley.com/go/shifflet/improvinghealthcarequality1e

avoidable preoperative delays that cause the date of surgery to be postponed. A rescheduled surgery not only increases overall healthcare cost but also wastes the time of the patient, scheduler, and doctor. Unused surgery time slots due to rescheduling may not be filled further delaying other surgeries. The hospital loses revenue by not having an effective system to efficiently complete all necessary prerequisites for TJRs.

13.5 The Task

Identify potential causes of avoidable preoperative delays and surgery reschedules through data analysis. In deepening the understanding of the preoperative process for the particular case of knee replacements, further data needed to be collected and validated. The team sought to understand the reasons for variability within and between the types of prosthetics. The primary metric, as defined by the process improvement team, was the elapsed time of the preoperative TJR process. This measure not only includes the start date but also the dates of major process steps. The objective is to identify the process steps that were the most time-consuming and target them for improvement moving forward.

13.6 The Data: TJR.jmp

The data was collected from the hospital's electronic health records system and can be found in TJR.jmp. (This is the data file that was processed for analysis in Chapter 12.) The data set contains variables that characterize each of the preoperative process cases regarding the type of prosthetic, provider, the reason for visit, insurance company, whether the patient attended joint replacement training, whether the primary care provider (PCP) is a network or out-of-network provider, and if the surgery was rescheduled or not. Dates were collected at different points in the preoperative TJR process and was used to determine the total elapsed time. Variable definitions can be found in Table 12.1.

13.7 Data Management

Identifying additional variables that could affect the elapsed time of the preoperative TJR process was not simple. The problem that the team encountered was that not all data, such as the recorded dates and times of some major process steps, were automatically collected in the hospital's patient record system. Other pieces of data resided in local databases or in the physicians' work calendars, for instance rescheduled surgery dates. Thus, the process improvement team, with the support of staff members related to the corresponding process steps, had to retrieve data manually. Information collected from these other data repositories, for instance, the patient joint class attendance dates, were validated against the paper files. When combining data from different sources, it is critical to verify that both the operational definitions and measurement scales and methods are the same.

Some additional data processing is required for the analysis presented in this case. There were three different types of knee implants used: Conformis, Stryker, and Zimmer. However, at this hospital, there is only one doctor specialized in each type of knee implant, so the information about the doctor performing the surgery is equivalent to the information on type of implant. The team also had to differentiate patients that were getting this joint implant for the first time vs. those who were being readmitted or having a joint "refurbished." This distinction is important as the preoperative process changes for these two types of patients. The way to identify the type of patient from the health records system was by looking at DRG code (which stands for diagnosis-related group) (Centers for Medicare and Medicaid Services, 2008). The DRG code is used across the United States to categorize patients into groups based on the types of treatments and services provided by a hospital. The team further narrowed the project to first time knee replacements, thus all the data points that were not linked to a DRG of 470 were omitted for further analysis. To obtain the desired records, select Rows > Data Filter, highlight Final Drg and click Add. Click 470 and all rows with a Final Drg value of 470 will be highlighted, then select Tables > Subset to extract these records into a new data table. Note that the only types of implants associated with the knee replacements having a DRG of 470 are Conformis and Zimmer.

13.8   Analysis

In gaining a more complete understanding of the preoperative TJR process performance, the team stratified the elapsed time data by variables that were potential causes of delay. The first layer of analysis consisted of visualizing the process variability by type of implant. Dr. 1 only works with Zimmer implants, whereas Dr. 2 works with both Conformis and Stryker. Box plots are useful for visualizing the process spread. When different processes are plotted on the same graph, box plots facilitate the comparison of process behavior in terms of location and spread. As shown in Figure 13.1, Conformis exhibits a higher median value in the overall elapsed time of the preoperative process. When the team talked to Dr. 2's staff, they found out that Conformis requires an extra step, a magnetic resonance imaging (MRI) scan, before the date of surgery. There is also a six-week lead time to make

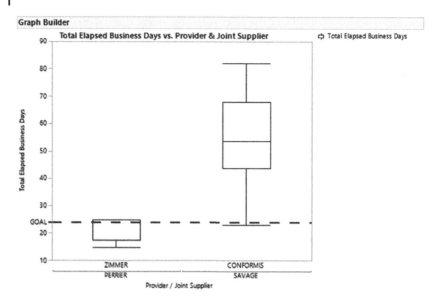

Figure 13.1 Box plots of Total Elapsed Business Days by type of knee implant. (Graph > Graph Builder. Drag "Total Elapsed Business Days" to the *y*-axis. Drag "Joint Supplier" to the *x*-Axis. Drag "Provider" to the *x*-axis under the joint supplier. Click on the box plot icon at the top. To add the reference line for the goal (at 24): Right click on any value on the *y*-axis > Axis Settings. In Reference Lines: For Value enter 24. In Label, enter "GOAL." Click "Done.")

each patient's custom Conformis prosthetic. This may explain a higher value in the elapsed time but does not necessarily explain the large variability in the process.

Reference lines can be added to the graph as shown in Figure 13.1. The dashed line is displayed at the goal set by the project team: 24 business days for the overall elapsed time for the preoperative process. While this graph gives an idea of the current capability of the process for meeting the target, the analysis can be enhanced by computing other statistics such as the coefficient of variation and other graphs as discussed later.

In comparing the variability of two different processes with different means, the CV has proved useful. CV is defined as the ratio of the standard deviation and the process mean, expressed as a percentage. The greater the percentage, the greater the variability relative to expected process behavior. Figure 13.2 shows the basic statistics used to compute the CV for the preoperative TJR processes of Conformis and Zimmer prosthetic implants. The differences in the relative variability are noticeable. For the Conformis case, the standard deviation is 32.44% of the expected elapsed time. Whereas for the Zimmer case, the standard deviation is 20.33% of the process mean. Even when the standard deviation is examined by

Tabulate

	Joint Supplier	Mean	Std Dev	CV
Days Between Scheduler Meeeting and Pre-op appt.	CONFORMIS	42.57	18.96	44.55
	ZIMMER	13.80	4.32	31.34
Days Between Pre-op appt and Pre-op clearance	CONFORMIS	3.07	1.64	53.37
	ZIMMER	4.20	2.77	66.07
Days between Pre-op Clearance and Surgery	CONFORMIS	9.43	4.94	52.41
	ZIMMER	6.00	2.65	44.10
Total Elapsed Business Days	CONFORMIS	53.07	17.22	32.44
	ZIMMER	22.00	4.47	20.33

Figure 13.2 Coefficient of variation of the preoperative TJR process (knee implant and 470 DRG code only). (Analyze > Tabulate. Multiple select the statistics: Mean, Std Dev, and CV and drag to the "Drop Zone for Columns." Next, multiple select: "Days between Scheduler Meeting and Pre-op appt," "Days Between Pre-op appt and Pre-op Clearance," "Days between Pre-op Clearance and Surgery," and "Total Elapsed Business Days." Drag the selected columns to the "Drop Zone for Rows." Drag "Joint Supplier" to the right of the first column (i.e. Joint Supplier will be in second column of the table). To format values with two decimal points: Select "Change Format." In Format check "Use the same decimal format." Set the format to "Fixed Dec" with two decimals. Click "OK." Click "Done.")

process steps, the differences between these two types of prosthetic implants are still noticeable. For instance, the CV of the elapsed time between the first consultation when the patient meets with the scheduler and the preoperative appointment is 44.55% for Conformis and 31.34% for Zimmer implants. Interestingly, the process step that exhibits more variability for both implant types, Conformis and Zimmer, is between the preoperative appointment and the clearance received. The difference in the CVs between Conformis and Zimmer suggests the need for further investigation as there might be other differentiating factors or process steps.

The second layer of analysis consisted of assessing whether the process was capable of meeting performance expectations. This is determined through a process capability study. The process capability analysis presented here is only considering a snapshot of the process as the data collected does not necessarily reflect the order in which patients were seen by the doctor. The process capability measure is a ratio that compares the amount of spread (or variability) of the process relative to the acceptable range of operation. A target value and tolerance range (expressed as a lower and upper specification limit [USL]) determine what constitutes an acceptable range of operation for the customer, or patient. In this case, the main concern was with the USL as it represented the amount of time a patient had to wait for their surgery. The USL was set at 45 business days due to the six-week lead time the suppliers need to get the customized Conformis prosthetic and the target was set to 24 days. The industry standard for an existing process sets a value of 1.33 to indicate that a process is capable of delivering an output (or in this case having

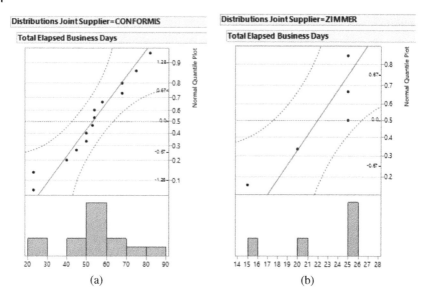

(a)   (b)

Figure 13.3 Histograms and normality tests for the elapsed times by type of knee implant: (a) Conformis and (b) Zimmer.
(Analyze > Distribution. From the Distribution dropdown menu select Stack. Select "Total Elapsed Business Days" and click Y, Columns. Select "Joint Supplier" and click "By." At the bottom left of the panel, check "Histograms Only." Click OK. From the Distribution dropdown menu select Stack. For Conformis: From the red triangle next to "Total Elapsed Business Days" select "Display Options" > "Summary Statistics." Click again on the red triangle next to "Total Elapsed Business Days" and select "Normal Quantile Plot." Repeat the above for "Zimmer.")

patients complete the preoperative process) within the specified range of operation set by the leadership team.

However, the process capability measure is not valid if the data is not normally distributed. As seen in Figure 13.3, the sample sizes of both the Conformis and Zimmer knee implants are relatively small, making it challenging to establish normality. The data points fall within the upper and lower confidence curves on the normal probability plot satisfying the normality assumption. The reader is referred to Kanji (1999) and SAS Institute (2018) for a more detailed discussion of normality and goodness-of-fit tests. The process improvement team proceeded with the capability analysis as it was evident that all patients requiring a Zimmer knee implant were consistently taking less than 45 days to complete the preoperative process.

Figure 13.4 shows the histograms with the target line and USL. Inspection of these two histograms indicates that the Conformis process mean is off-target and a disproportionate number of patients exceed the USL of 45 business days. Since we are only concerned with the USL, the Ppk capability ratio is calculated as the

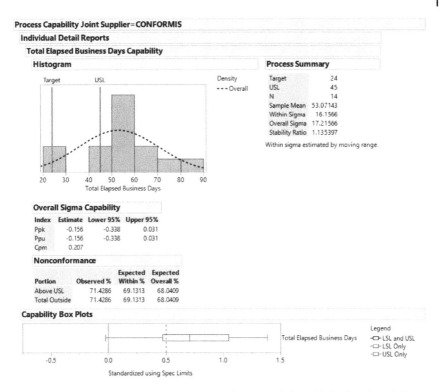

Process Capability Joint Supplier = CONFORMIS

Individual Detail Reports

Total Elapsed Business Days Capability

Histogram

Process Summary

Target	24
USL	45
N	14
Sample Mean	53.07143
Within Sigma	16.1566
Overall Sigma	17.21566
Stability Ratio	1.135397

Within sigma estimated by moving range.

Overall Sigma Capability

Index	Estimate	Lower 95%	Upper 95%
Ppk	-0.156	-0.338	0.031
Ppu	-0.156	-0.338	0.031
Cpm	0.207		

Nonconformance

Portion	Observed %	Expected Within %	Expected Overall %
Above USL	71.4286	69.1313	68.0409
Total Outside	71.4286	69.1313	68.0409

Capability Box Plots

Legend
-□- LSL and USL
-□- LSL Only
-□- USL Only

Standardized using Spec Limits

Figure 13.4   Capability ratios of the preoperative elapsed time: (a) Conformis and (b) Zimmer. (Analyze > Quality and Process > Process Capability. Select "Total Elapsed Business Days" and click "Y, Process." Select "Joint Supplier" and click "By." Click OK. In the Specification Limits dialog box input the Target of 24 and the USL of 45. Click OK. Use red arrows to make appropriate report selections.)

ratio of the difference (USL − mean) to three times the process standard deviation (overall sigma in Figure 13.4). For example, the Ppk for the Conformis implant is $(45 − 53.07)/51.65 = −0.156$. The Ppk gives an assessment of the overall process capability taking into account both the process location and variation. The higher the Ppk value, the more capable the process. This explains the negative value of the capability ratio (Ppk), where 72% of the patients taking longer than 45 business days. The scenario is different for patients requiring a Zimmer knee implant with a Ppk = 1.714, where the process mean is essentially at the targeted level of 24 business days and with zero cases taking longer than 45 business days. The Zimmer process is more capable compared to the Conformis process. Bear in mind that these process capability ratios are based on a small number of data points.

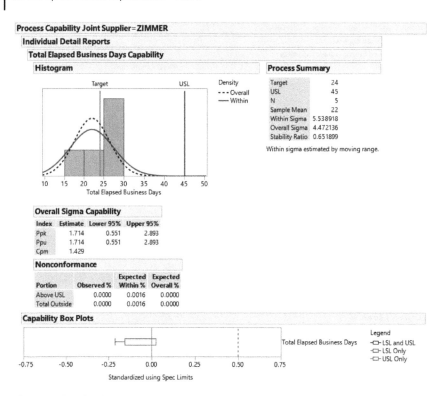

Figure 13.4 (*Continued*)

In investigating the differences in the preoperative process between these two types of prosthetics, the process improvement team mapped each process at a detailed level to identify sources of variation. After mapping the main process activities with the aid of a swimlane diagram and a fishbone diagram, the process improvement team and the hospital staff identified potential causes (or potential critical X's) of variability and long elapsed times of the preoperative process. These potential Xs are time of the year, patient initial health, order of scheduling appointments, orthopedic surgeon backlog, if the patient has a PCP and if so, if the PCP is within the hospital network or out-of-network, and type of prosthetic. As in Chapter 12, the variability greatly stemmed from the first day of consultation, that is, when the patient met with the scheduler, and the PCP appointment. In looking closer at this process step, the process team realized that the appointment scheduling approach is different depending on the type of implant. The scheduling process is not standardized and this might be due to the fact that there is one dedicated scheduler for each type of implant (i.e. one scheduler for Conformis and another scheduler for Zimmer.) The scheduling process for patients in need of a Conformis prosthetic starts by booking the surgery date and then works backward to book the PCP appointment. Whereas for patients in need of a Zimmer prosthetic, the scheduling process starts by booking the PCP appointment first and then works forward to choose the date of surgery. Given the difference in the approaches, the process improvement team was interested in identifying if the scheduling approach could be considered a statistically significant source of variability. The team decided to conduct a hypothesis test comparing total elapsed time between the two implant types, which is discussed in Chapter 14.

13.9 Summary

13.9.1 Statistical Insights

At this stage of the DMAIC methodology, the process improvement team identified factors (or process inputs) associated with the variability in elapsed days in the preoperative TJR process. Some of the process inputs are beyond the control of the hospital; for example, the initial patient health stage or the patient's preference of having a PCP within the hospital's network. While these variables certainly affect the overall elapsed time, the focus for further statistical analysis should be on the input variables for which the hospital has control. In deepening the understanding of the process behavior, process capability analysis has proved insightful despite the small sample sizes. The team continued to collect data as it became available. Moreover, one of the main difficulties in quality improvement projects applied to healthcare is that, more often than not, the process under study is being measured in a new or different way. Not surprisingly, there are cases, like in this project, where even the acceptable performance level is not set for a particular project metric. Thus, the process improvement team was faced with the challenge of setting a reasonable and acceptable target level or range for operation. These values matter as they serve as a reference from which the process data is evaluated against this specification. Thus, unrealistic specifications may mislead the process capability analysis and give the wrong signals to the team. Therefore, the team discussed the target and USLs with the process experts, that is, the people who do the job and the orthopedics practice manager.

At the Measure and Analyze stages of the project, the process improvement team faced the challenge of first obtaining the data necessary for detailed analyses. Oftentimes, all of the data is not in a single repository and must be retrieved from multiple sources and then formatted and prepared for statistical analysis. Data acquisition and preparation are often more time-consuming than anticipated. Misleading conclusions can result from a good analysis conducted on flawed data. Another challenge the process improvement team faced had to do with the actual performance measurement of the preoperative TJR process by type of knee implants. In addition to establishing a realistic (and acceptable) performance level, sample sizes collected were relatively small, making it harder to obtain conclusive results, such as the case with the normality testing for the Zimmer knee implant. Nevertheless, the team measured the process spread against the process specification to assess the process capability for both types of knees' implants.

13.9.2 Implications and Next Steps

The objective of the next statistical analysis should be on understanding to what extent each of the potential sources of variation (Xs) affects the elapsed time, and what values should be set for these process inputs to minimize the effect of the other uncontrollable process input variables. With this in mind, the team will further analyze the few critical X's from which ideas for improvement will be generated.

13.9.3 Summary of Tools and JMP Features

Statistical methods tools	Data management concepts	JMP platform features	Quality tools
Data visualization	Subsetting	Graph builder	Process variation
– Box plots			
– Histograms			
– Normal probability plot			
Descriptive statistics		Distribution	Root cause
Coefficient of variation		Quality and process	Process capability
Process capability analysis			

13.9.4 Exercises

1. Using the data found in TJR.jmp, conduct a capability analysis for the elapsed time of the preoperative process for hip replacements, in particular for the Stryker type of implant.

   (a) Is the data for the Stryker hip replacement normally distributed?

   (b) Is the preoperative process capable of helping patients go through the process in less than 45 days?

2. Select another variable that may be a potential cause of delay in the preoperative surgery process and repeat the analysis shown in this case. What do you conclude from this analysis?
3. Cpk is another process capability measure useful in quality improvement. Consult some books, articles, or websites to help you answer the following questions:
   (a) How is Cpk defined and calculated? Cite your references.
   (b) Using the data from this case calculate Cpk for knee replacements only.
   (c) Compare the Cpk to Ppk. What is the difference between Cpk and Ppk?
   (d) Which process capability measure do you think is most appropriate for this case? Explain your reasoning.

13.9.5 Discussion Questions

1. The process improvement team invested a significant amount of time and effort in identifying potential causes of delay for their analyses. Why was this important and how could that have affected their course of action?
2. The process improvement team had to collect data from different sources such as provider's schedules, electronic health records, logs, etc. Do you think this was particular to this hospital or is it something commonly found in healthcare organizations? Do you think data is available to depict the overall process or fragmented or in silos? Discuss how data is maintained and organized in a healthcare organization you are familiar with.
3. The process capability analysis is based on the normality assumption. There are different normality tests. Investigate the different types of normality tests and identify situations for which each is appropriate.
4. One of the challenges in determining the process capability is defining the acceptable range of operation. Identify and discuss the different approaches that can be used to establish process targets.

References

Centers for Medicare and Medicaid Services (2008). List of Diagnosis Related Groups (DRGs). http://cms.gov (accessed 28 August 2019).

Kanji, G.K. (1999). *100 Statistical Tests*. Sage Publications.

SAS Institute (2018). JMP®14 Basic Analysis. https://support.sas.com/documentation/onlinedoc/jmp/14.0/Basic-Analysis.pdf (accessed 1 August 2019).

14

Pre-Op TJR Process Improvement – Part 3

14.1   Key Concepts

Hypothesis testing, two sample *t*-test, equality of variance test, data visualization.

14.2   DMAIC

I: The tools illustrated in this case are frequently applied in the Improve phase of the Define–Measure–Analyze–Improve–Control (DMAIC) approach to process improvement.

14.3   PDCA

C: The tools illustrated in this case are frequently applied in the Check step of the Plan–Do–Check–Act (PDCA) approach to process improvement.

14.4   Background

In Chapter 13, the process improvement team learned that there were differences in the elapsed times of the preoperative total joint replacement (TJR) process. The team then identified the sources (or factors) that might explain the differences observed in the process variability. Among those factors, the process improvement team was particularly interested in the type of knee implant needed by the patient. Patients could either have a Zimmer or Conformis prosthetic. The type of knee implant chosen depends on a variety of factors including patient age, weight, lifestyle, and degree of joint deterioration. As discovered by the team, the Conformis prosthetic required an magnetic resonance imaging (MRI) scan

Improving Health Care Quality: Case Studies with JMP®, First Edition.
Mary Ann Shifflet, Cecilia Martinez, Jane Oppenlander, and Shirley Shmerling.
© 2020 John Wiley & Sons, Inc. Published 2020 by John Wiley & Sons, Inc.
Books Companion site:www.wiley.com/go/shifflet/improvinghealthcarequality1e

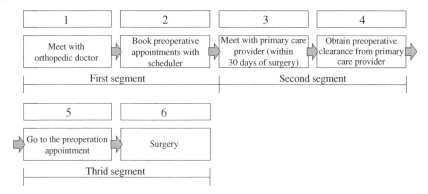

Figure 14.1 Preoperative TJR process segmentation.

and several weeks to order a custom-made prosthetic. Thereby, the preoperative expected elapsed time was longer for patients needing a Conformis prosthetic than the elapsed time for patients requiring a Zimmer implant. The differences in the process variability were even more evident when the process was broken down into three segments: from the initial consultation/scheduler meeting to the primary care provider (PCP) appointment, from the PCP appointment to the preoperative clearance, and from the preoperative clearance to surgery (see Figure 14.1). However, it was not known if these differences were statistically significant. That is, the process improvement team still needed to know whether there was sufficient difference in the elapsed times between the groups to be considered more than simply usual variability. To this aim, an analysis was conducted to determine the extent to which these sources of variability affected the process elapsed time.

14.5 The Task

Evaluate the effect of implant type on elapsed time of the preoperative TJR process to determine if the observed difference is statistically lower for Zimmer than for Conformis. From the insights gained, the process improvement team will be better positioned for identifying and validating the most critical causal relationships. Then, the team could proceed to brainstorm ideas for improving the elapsed preoperative time of such causal relationships and drive the process performance to the desired level.

14.6 The Data: TJR.jmp

The data was collected from the hospital's electronic health records system and can be found in TJR.jmp. (This is the data file that was used in Chapters 12 and 13.) The data set contains variables that characterize the preoperative process case including the type of prosthetic, provider, the reason for visit, insurance company, whether the patient attended joint replacement training, whether the PCP is a network or out-of-network provider, and if the surgery was rescheduled or not. Dates were also collected at different points in the preoperative TJR process and were aggregated to determine the total elapsed time. The variables are defined in Table 12.1.

14.7 Data Management

No further processing is required for the data contained in TJR.jmp to conduct the analyses presented in this case.

14.8 Analysis

To familiarize themselves with the difference in total elapsed time for the two different knee implant types, a dot plot, as shown in Figure 14.2, was created. This

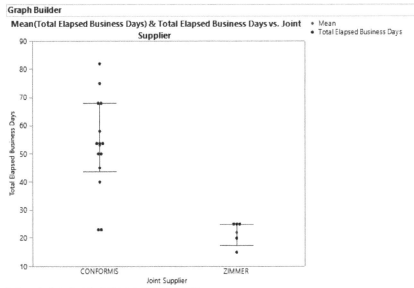

Figure 14.2 Dot plot for elapsed times of the TJR knee implants.
(Graph > Graph Builder. Drag "Total Elapsed Business Days" to the y-axis. Drag "Joint Supplier" to the x-Axis. On the left panel titled "Points": For "Summary Statistics" select "Mean." For "Error Bars" select "Interquartile Range." Right click anywhere on the graph. Select "Add" > "Points." Click "Done.")

plot offers an easy way to quickly assess differences in the center and variability in total elapsed time by knee implant. There appears to be more variability and generally longer total elapsed time for the Conformis implant compared to the Zimmer implant.

Numerical estimates of the average level of performance and variability will provide a more detailed comparison of the process time associated with the two implant types. Figure 14.3 shows histograms and descriptive statistics obtained from the JMP® Distribution platform. Note that the histograms have been placed on a common *x*-axis scale. This is important for accurate visual comparison.

The difference in the mean total elapsed times is approximately 31 days longer for Conformis implants compared to Zimmer implants. While this difference appears large, it is important to establish whether it is statistically significant, meaning that the difference is due to something other than sampling error.

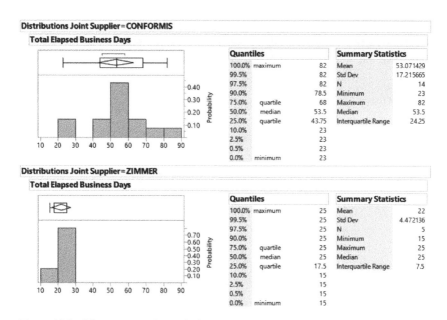

Figure 14.3 Histograms and descriptive statistics for total elapsed time by implant type. (Analyze > Distribution. Enter "Total Elapsed Business Days" in the Y, Columns field and Joint Supplier in the By field. Hold <ctrl> and select Customize Summary Statistics from the Summary Statistics dropdown menu. Continue holding <ctrl> and select Mean, Std Dev, N, Minimum, Maximum, Median, and Interquartile Range. Click OK. <ctrl> click and select Uniform Scaling from the Distributions Joint Supplier = Conformis dropdown menu.)

Sampling error is the uncertainty associated with a sample estimate to the extent that it is not a complete representation of the whole population or process.

An analysis tool commonly used in the Improve stage of DMAIC is hypothesis testing. Hypothesis testing is a statistical inference method that determines if sample evidence is consistent with a posed hypothesis. When two independent groups are to be compared, a two sample *t*-test can be applied which allows us to determine if there is a statistically significant relationship between an independent (explanatory or input) variable (e.g. the type of knee implant) and a continuous variable (e.g. the process elapsed time). This will help the project team establish if the type of implant has a causal relationship with elapsed time. When more than two groups are to be compared, analysis of variance (ANOVA) is an appropriate method. For additional details on statistical inference and hypothesis testing, see Polit (2010) and Rosner (2015).

To determine if the observed difference in the total elapsed times is due to sampling error (or chance), the difference in implant means is compared to the standard error of that difference. The standard error is a measure of precision associated with a sample statistic, i.e. how much variability there is in the estimate. There are two forms of the two sample *t*-test, one that assumes the variances of the two groups are equal and another that assumes the variances of the two groups are not equal. As shown in Figure 14.2, the preoperative TJR process time appears more variable for patients requiring a Conformis prosthetic; the process improvement team suspected the two groups have unequal variances. As a first step, an equality (or homogeneity) of variance test should be conducted.

Figure 14.4 shows the results from several different equality of variance tests. The graph shows the values of the standard deviations are 17.22 and 4.47 for the Conformis and Zimmer prosthetics, respectively. The null hypothesis associated with these tests is that the variances of the two groups are equal vs. the alternative hypothesis that they are not equal.

The various tests for comparing variances have different assumptions. For example, Bartlett's test and the *F*-test are sensitive to the normality assumption, while the Levene test is less sensitive. Still, these results need to be interpreted with caution due to the small sample sizes. (Note the warning statement under the test results in Figure 14.4.) Looking at Figure 14.3, we see that the distribution of the Conformis elapsed times is relatively bell-shaped, however, the distribution of Zimmer is not. With such small sample sizes, establishing normality (or any other distribution) can be difficult. Therefore, we will use the Levene test for comparing the variances, which yields a *p*-value of 0.1039; therefore, we can assume that the variances of the two implant groups are equal. Further detail on the equality of variance tests can be found in SAS Institute (2018).

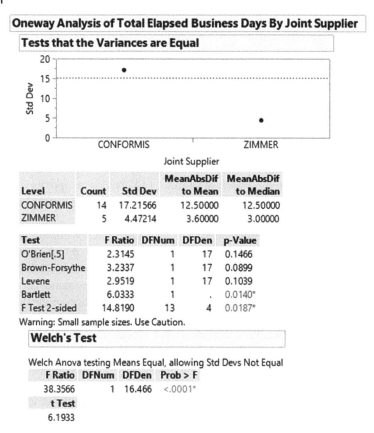

Oneway Analysis of Total Elapsed Business Days By Joint Supplier

Tests that the Variances are Equal

Level	Count	Std Dev	MeanAbsDif to Mean	MeanAbsDif to Median
CONFORMIS	14	17.21566	12.50000	12.50000
ZIMMER	5	4.47214	3.60000	3.00000

Test	F Ratio	DFNum	DFDen	p-Value
O'Brien[.5]	2.3145	1	17	0.1466
Brown-Forsythe	3.2337	1	17	0.0899
Levene	2.9519	1	17	0.1039
Bartlett	6.0333	1	.	0.0140*
F Test 2-sided	14.8190	13	4	0.0187*

Warning: Small sample sizes. Use Caution.

Welch's Test

Welch Anova testing Means Equal, allowing Std Devs Not Equal

F Ratio	DFNum	DFDen	Prob > F
38.3566	1	16.466	<.0001*

t Test
6.1933

Figure 14.4 Equality of variance tests for Total Elapsed Business Days by Joint Supplier. (Analyze > Fit Y by X. Select "Total Elapsed Business Days" and click "Y, Process." Select "Joint Supplier" and click "X, Factor." Click OK. Click red triangle next to "Oneway Analysis of Total Elapsed Time By Joint Supplier" and select "Unequal Variances." To remove the graph click again on the red triangle next to "Oneway analysis of Total Elapsed Time by Joint Supplier," select "Display Options," and deselect "All Graphs.")

Having established that the variances of the total elapsed time for the two implant groups are equal, the project team proceeded to conduct a two sample t-test with equal variances. The null hypothesis is that the means of the two implant types are the same with the alternative hypothesis that the means are different. This test will determine if the difference of 31 days is statistically significant or not. Figure 14.5 shows the results for the two-sample t-test.

The JMP output displays "Oneway Anova" in the heading. This is because the Fit Y by X platform is used for both the two sample t-test and the one-way ANOVA; JMP displays the appropriate output based on the number of groups detected in the

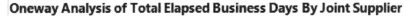

Oneway Analysis of Total Elapsed Business Days By Joint Supplier

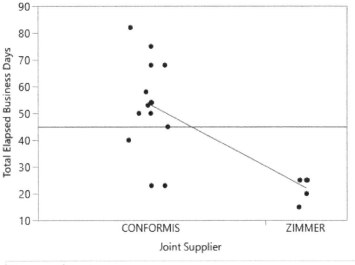

Oneway Anova

Pooled t Test

ZIMMER-CONFORMIS
Assuming equal variances

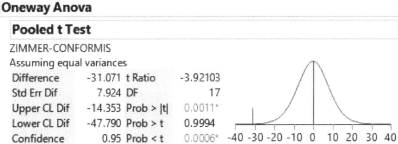

Difference	-31.071	t Ratio	-3.92103
Std Err Dif	7.924	DF	17
Upper CL Dif	-14.353	Prob > |t|	0.0011*
Lower CL Dif	-47.790	Prob > t	0.9994
Confidence	0.95	Prob < t	0.0006*

Figure 14.5 *t*-Test of Total Elapsed Business Days by Joint Supplier. (Analyze > Fit Y by X. Select "Total Elapsed Business Days" and click "Y, Process." Select "Joint Supplier" and click "X, Factor." Click OK. Click red triangle next to "Oneway Analysis of Total Elapsed Time By Joint Supplier" and select "Means/Anova/Pooled t." Click again on the red triangle and choose Display Options and check All Graphs, Points, Grand Mean, Connect Means, X Axis Proportional, Points Jittered, and Legend.)

independent variable (X) column. The points on the graph have been "jittered" to better visualize the distribution of elapsed times and the means of the two groups have been connected to more easily assess the difference in the implant means visually.

At the beginning of the Pooled *t*-Test output, the order of the difference is given. By default, the first alphabetical group is subtracted from the second alphabetical group. The order of the subtraction can be changed with the Value Ordering column property found in the Column Information associated with the Joint

Supplier column. The Pooled *t*-Test output gives the estimated difference in total elapsed time for the implant type means and the associated 95% confidence interval (Upper CL dif and Lower CL dif). The 95% confidence interval is [−47.8, −14.4] days which is interpreted as a range of plausible values for the true mean process difference. The key result for a hypothesis test is the *p*-value; three possible *p*-values are displayed in the JMP output (Prob >|*t*|, Prob >*t*, and Prob <*t*). These correspond to the three possible alternative hypotheses, that the means are different, the mean of Zimmer is greater than the mean of Conformis, and the mean of Zimmer is less than the mean of Conformis. Only one alternative hypothesis should be chosen when the hypothesis test is set up and it should correspond to the research question posed. In this case, the alternative hypothesis is that the mean elapsed time for Zimmer is smaller than for Conformis, therefore, the Prob <*t* = 0.0006 is the appropriate *p*-value. The *p*-value is defined on a scale of 0–1 where small *p*-values cause a rejection of the null hypothesis and large *p*-values support the null hypothesis. The *p*-value is the likelihood of obtaining the sample difference in means or something more extreme assuming the null hypothesis is true. The null hypothesis is rejected since the *p*-value is less than 0.05, the chosen significance level. The significance level is the risk of incorrectly rejecting the null hypothesis and is chosen when the hypothesis test is set up. The hypothesis test shows us that the mean elapsed time of the preoperative TJR process for Zimmer is significantly less than for Conformis by 31 business days.

With this significant difference, the process improvement team wanted to investigate whether this pattern was present throughout the entire preoperative process or was due to a particular process step. The team then conducted *t*-tests for the three process segments shown in Figure 14.1. Figure 14.6 gives the results of the equal variances test for each process segment and first shows the dot plot for each subprocess (the observations have not been jittered). In looking at these graphs, the spread of the observations for the first process segment, that is, from the initial consultation and meeting with the scheduler to the PCP appointment, are noticeably different. The Levene test does not support this impression with a *p*-value of 0.1020, so we conclude that for this first segment, the variances are equal of the two implant types. This reinforces the importance of hypothesis testing to establish statistical significance rather than subjective visual impressions. For the other two segments, the Levene test also finds that the two implant types have equal variances.

Figure 14.7 displays the *t*-test with equal variances output for the three process segments. The results are summarized in Table 14.1. Extracting the important results from the JMP output and presenting them in tabular form assists the project team and stakeholders in easily assimilating the information.

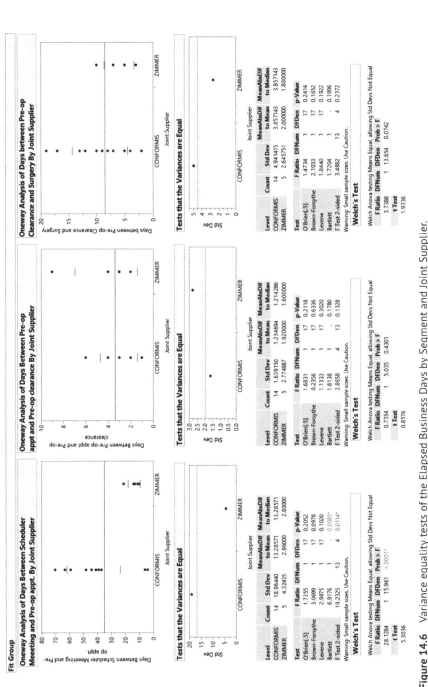

Figure 14.6 Variance equality tests of the Elapsed Business Days by Segment and Joint Supplier.
(Analyze > Fit Y by X. Multiple select "Days between Scheduler Meeting and Pre-op appt," "Days Between Pre-op appt and Pre-op Clearance," "Days Between Pre-op Clearance and Surgery," and click "Y, Response." Select "Joint Supplier" and click "X, Factor." Click OK. Click on the red triangle next to "Oneway analysis of Total Elapsed Time by Joint Supplier" and select "Unequal Variances.")

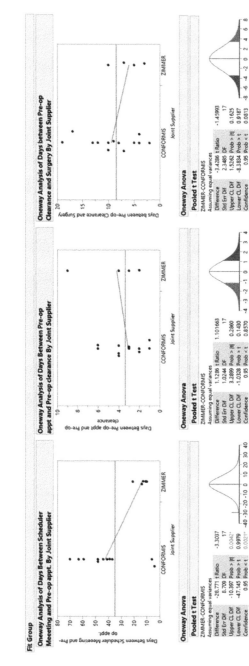

Figure 14.7 *t*-Tests for each TJR preoperative process segment.

(Analyze > Fit Y by X. Multiple select "Days between Scheduler Meeting and Pre-op appt," "Days Between Pre-op appt and Pre-op Clearance," "Days Between Pre-op Clearance and Surgery," and click "Y, Response." Select "Joint Supplier" and click "X, Factor." Click OK. <ctrl> click on the red triangle next to "Oneway analysis of Days Between Scheduler Meeting and Pre-op appt by Joint Supplier" and select "Means/Anova/Pooled t." <ctrl> click again on the red triangle and choose Display Options and check All Graphs, Points, Grand Mean, Connect Means, X Axis Proportional, Points Jittered, and Legend.)

Table 14.1 Summary of *t*-tests for process segments.

Segment	Delay days between	Difference in Means Zimmer–Conformis	*p*-value	95% CI for difference in means
1	Scheduler meeting and pre-op appt	−28.8	0.0021	[−42.1, −10.4]
2	Pre-op appt and pre-op clearance	1.1	0.8570	[−1.0, 3.3]
3	Pre-op clearance and surgery	−3.4	0.0813	[−8.4, 1.5]

From Table 14.1, we see that only the first segment, the time between the scheduler meeting and preoperative appointment is the average time for Zimmer significantly lower than the average time for Conformis. The differences in means between the implant types are not significant for the other two segments. Those differences observed are due to sampling error.

14.9 Summary

14.9.1 Statistical Insights

The use of statistical inference in the Improve phase of the project allowed the project team to discover significant differences in the total elapsed time for the two different types of knee implants. Establishing statistical significance indicates when meaningful differences have occurred, rather than being just due to chance. All too often, actions are taken without verifying statistical significance and this may lead to wasted resources and changes that do not actually improve the process. In this case, the tests were conducted before process changes were implemented. This can assist the project team in narrowing the scope of the project or prioritizing improvement efforts. Statistical inference methods are also commonly used to verify that the changes in the process were effective.

When interpreting the results of a significant hypothesis test, it is important to assess the magnitude of the outcome in practical terms. The difference of 31 days seems to be substantial and worthy of continued improvement effort. Had the difference been considerably smaller, say one day, this might not be a large enough difference to warrant further attention. It is important to interpret statistical results in the problem context.

The two sample *t*-tests shown here are valid when the assumption of equal variances is met. If this assumption is not met, a *t*-test for unequal variances should be used instead. This *t*-test can be executed in JMP from Analyze > Fit Y by X >*t*-test. When comparing means for more than two groups, one-way ANOVA is the appropriate method.

14.9.2 Implications and Next Steps

The results indicated that if the average number of business days between the scheduler meeting and the PCP preoperative meeting are reduced, the total average number of business days for the entire preoperative process can be brought down drastically to the baseline requirements. During discussions, the process improvement team had to identify root causes for the lengthy preoperative delay. While creating the fishbone diagram, the team discovered that different scheduling approaches (e.g. booking the surgery date and then working backward vs. booking the PCP appointment and then working forward) were used for the preoperative appointments and surgery. The analysis results indicated that the difference in scheduling approaches does result in a statistical difference in the elapsed times of the preoperative process. Patients in need of a Conformis knee replacement consistently experienced larger elapsed time averages and more variation than patients in need of a Zimmer knee replacement. When the scheduler for Conformis patients was asked why she used a backward approach (surgery date is scheduled first), she said that it was due to patient load. According to her, she had to start with the surgery date because if scheduled working forward, she would land on a surgery date that was not available because the provider was already booked. Guided by this input, the process improvement team wanted to explore this explanation in more detail.

Surprisingly, when the team looked at the number of surgery days each surgeon had available each quarter, along with the number of surgeries they could perform in one day and compared this to the patient demand, the team found that the surgeons actually had very similar patient loads. In fact, both of them had about three surgery days per quarter that were being unused.

Through this quality improvement initiative, it was discovered that there was no clear process that schedulers should adhere to when setting up appointments for patients. If a standardized set of steps were implemented the number of skipped appointments and waiting times between appointments could be reduced. One potential solution included switching the order that appointments were scheduled, matching available surgery days to patient load, preventing patients from meeting with the scheduler until they have acquired a PCP, preventing patients from meeting with the scheduler unless they have their insurance information, identifying patients that are going to need a specialist consult during the scheduler meeting, and creating the appointment with the scheduler.

Variation in this preoperative TJR process ultimately occurs because every patient is different. There is no "one size fits all" solution to making each patient's experience exactly the same. However, the root causes of added time in the interval between the scheduler meeting and the PCP preoperative appointment can be narrowed down to a handful of factors. Among those are the consideration of some patients having insurance and only some having PCPs. Other root causes include some patients having availability issues on certain dates that get in the way of appointments, and some patients needing extra tests done (Conformis CT scan and lab screenings) before surgeries can be performed. Another root cause includes the order in which the scheduler makes patient's appointments. By starting with the next closest appointment, variation is proven to be reduced in Zimmer's processes. Every patient cannot be scheduled exactly the same way, but by minimizing the effects of these root causes as soon as possible in the process and by having set workarounds for them, waste can be eliminated and patients can get through the process more quickly and consistently.

The process improvement team proposed a solution of scheduling appointments closest to the present first, rather than starting with a defined surgery date and working back. In addition to this, better patient communication about the importance of appointment dates and having insurance information ready was also recommended. The next step of the DMAIC is to evaluate the effectiveness of the potential solution in the process, however, data is not yet available for such an analysis.

Overall, the results of this project brought a number of benefits to the hospital, including better operating room utilization. By making the scheduling process more standardized and less prone to reschedules, fewer surgery time slots were missed and left open. By having fewer open surgery time slots, the hospital was able to more efficiently use both surgeon and operating room availability. Orthopedic surgeons were able to see more patients and operate more often. Another benefit is that less employee time was used to reschedule appointments. If fewer patients are missing or canceling appointments, the schedulers, nurses, and doctors spend less of their valuable time reworking appointment schedules in order to accommodate patients. Lastly, patients have a much higher degree of satisfaction when they are able to get through the process quicker. By doing this, they spend less time living in unbearable pain and as a result, will be much happier with the hospital's services.

14.9.3 Summary of Tools and JMP Features

Statistical methods tools	Data management concepts	JMP platform features	Quality tools
Data visualization		Graph builder	Sources of variation
– *Dot plots*			
Confidence intervals		Distribution	Root cause
Equal variance tests		Fit Y by X	
Two sample *t*-test			

14.9.4 Exercises

1. The process improvement team focused only on patients requiring a knee implant for the first time. That is, only patient records with the final diagnosis-related group (DRG) code 470 were considered for analysis. Conduct an analysis to evaluate whether there is a significant difference in the overall elapsed time between patients requiring a total knee implant vs. a refurbished implant.

2. Create a dot plot of the total elapsed business days for all the pairwise subgroups that result from combining the different insurance companies and the type of knee implant. What do you learn from this plot?

3. When comparing the means of more than two groups, one-way ANOVA is an appropriate analysis technique.

   (a) To learn how to conduct a one-way ANOVA, review the JMP Many Means Tutorial which can be found from Help > Tutorial > Many Means Tutorial.

   (b) Use the JMP Fit Model platform to perform a one-way ANOVA to see if there is a significant effect of month on the total elapsed time for patients requiring a new knee implant.

   (c) Give some possible reasons that might explain the results from the one-way ANOVA conducted in part (b).

4. Explore the concept of effect size. Write a brief summary of your findings and cite your sources. Explain how effect size is helpful in a quality improvement project. How would knowing effect size be useful in the TJR case?

14.9.5 Discussion Questions

1. What is the difference between a two sample *t*-test and a test of the difference in the means using confidence intervals? When would be more appropriate to use one or the another? Cite some examples, where each type of *t*-test is applicable.
2. Empirical evidence alone is generally not sufficient for establishing causality. Search the Internet to find the Bradford Hill causality criteria. Discuss which of these criteria are applicable in the TJR process. Suggest ways in which the applicable criteria could be satisfied.
3. Another process analysis tool is the χ^2 analysis. Investigate the basics of this type of analysis and discuss in what ways it differs from ANOVA. When would be more appropriate to use one or the another? Explain.
4. Do a literature review to identify published quality improvement projects involving preoperative processes. Discuss your findings and how they compare with this case.
5. Find an article that describes a study in a field of interest to you where effect size is reported. Give a summary of the study and explain what the effect size tells you about the study results.

References

Polit, D.F. (2010). *Statistics and Data Analysis for Nursing Research*, 2e. Pearson.

Rosner, B. (2015). *Fundamentals of Biostatistics*, 8e. Cengage Learning.

SAS Institute (2018). JMP®14 Basic Analysis. https://support.sas.com/documentation/onlinedoc/jmp/14.0/Basic-Analysis.pdf (accessed 1 August 2019).

Index

Printed and bound by CPI Group (UK) Ltd, Croydon, CR0 4YY

16/04/2025